Organon of Homoeopathic Medicine

*The Classic Guide Book for Understanding Homeopathy
– the Fifth and Sixth Edition Texts, with Notes*

By Samuel Hahnemann

*Translated by R. E. Dudgeon (5th Edition)
and William Boericke (6th Edition)*

PANTIANOS
CLASSICS

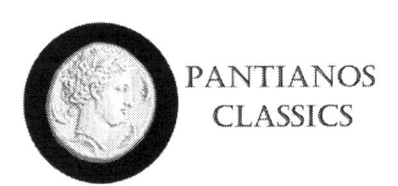

Published by Pantianos Classics

ISBN-13: 978-1729809662

First published in 1836

This edition is adapted from the English translations of 1893 and 1922

Contents

Translator's Preface .... *iv*
Introduction .... *vi*
Author's Preface to the Sixth Edition .... *xi*
Introduction .... *xiv*
The Aphorisms **33**
Notes **124**

Translator's Preface

The sixth edition of the "Organon" as left by Hahnemann ready for publication, was found to be an interleaved copy of the fifth, the last German edition, published in 1833. In his eighty-sixth year, while in active practice in Paris, he completed the thorough revision of it by carefully going over paragraph by paragraph, making changes, erasures, annotations and additions.

Hahnemann himself had apprized several friends of the preparation of another edition of his great work as is evident among other from a letter to Boenninghausen, his most appreciative follower and intimate friend. Writing to him from Paris, he states: "I am at work on the sixth edition of the 'Organon,' to which I devote several hours on Sundays and Thursdays, all the other time being required for treatment of patients who come to my rooms." And to his publisher, Mr. Schaub, in Dusseldorf, he wrote in a letter dated Paris, February 20, 1842: "I have now, after eighteen months of work, finished the sixth edition of my 'Organon,' the most nearly perfect of all." He further expressed the wish to have it printed in the best possible style as regards paper, perfectly new type and in short desired its appearance to be unexceptionally fine as it would most likely be the last. These wishes of the venerable author have been carried out perfectly by the present publishers.

All these annotations, changes, and addition I have carefully translated from the original copy in my possession. Hahnemann made these in his own wonderfully small, clear handwriting, perfectly preserved during all these years and as legible today as when first written. For those extensive parts in which he made no changes whatever, including his long Introduction, I have adopted Dr. Dudgeon's fine translation of the fifth edition, which has the distinction of perfect English with a remarkable, faithful adherence to the peculiar Hahnemannian style and setting.

The following are some of the more important changes noted in this final edition.

In a long footnote to Paragraph 11 he gives a consideration of the important question: What is dynamic influence – dynamis – and in Paragraphs 22 and 29 will be found his last views on the life principle, which term he uses throughout, preferably to vital force as in former editions.

Paragraphs 52 to 56 have been wholly rewritten and long footnotes are added to Paragraphs 60-74. Again, Paragraph 148 is practically wholly new and concerns itself with the origin of disease, denying a *materia peccans*, as the prime etiological factor.

Of greatest importance are Paragraphs 246-248 in regard to dosage in the treatment of chronic diseases. He there departs from the single dose and advises repetition of dosage but in different potencies. Paragraphs 269-272 are devoted to technical directions for the preparation of homoeopathic medicines especially according to his latest views.

The vexed question of double remedies other than chemical compounds is fully and definitely settled in Paragraph 273 and all doubts as to the impropriety of, such procedure removed.

Wholly new is the footnote to Paragraph 282 and of greatest importance. Here his treatment of the chronic diseases under psora, syphilis, and sycosis departs absolutely from that advised in former editions. He now advises to commence treatment with large doses of their specific remedies early and, if necessary, several times daily and gradually ascend to higher degrees of dynamization. In the treatment of figwarts, local application is considered necessary with the internal use of the remedy.

The book as now presented is Hahnemann's last work concerning the principles advanced by him in the first and subsequent editions, illuminated and enlarged by his vast experience in the latter part of his medical career in the treatment of both acute and chronic diseases. Historically, the book in its sixth edition is of greatest interest and importance, completing as it does the marvellous array of Hahnemann's philosophic insight into the practice of medicine. Hahnemann's "Organon" is the high water mark of medical philosophy, the practical interpretation of which produces a veritable mountain of light and will guide the physician by means of the Law of Cure to a new world in therapeutics.

This edition is favored with an introduction by Dr. James Krauss, of Boston, the learned and scholarly student of Hahnemann, to whom I herewith desire to express my grateful appreciation for both the introduction and other valuable aid.

William Boericke.
San Francisco, December, 1921.

Introduction

By James Krauss, M.D. Boston, September 30, 1921.
To Doctor Boericke's translation of the 6th edition of Hahnemann's "Organon."

The excellence of the Dudgeon translation into English of the fifth German edition of Hahnemann's "Organon" is thoroughly maintained throughout this English translation of the sixth German edition by Doctor William Boericke, to whom the medical profession is under a double debt for rescuing this last authentic work of Hahnemann from possible loss and for putting it into good, clear, unparaphrased English. Twice, this manuscript of Hahnemann was in danger of being lost, once during the siege of Paris in the Franco-Prussian war of 1870-71, and once in the military over-running of Westphalia during the World War of 1914-18. Doctor Boericke was the main instrument for procuring this last medical manuscript of Hahnemann for the medical world.

Everything that Hahnemann ever wrote is of historic medical interest, for notwithstanding all attempts of ignorant, prejudiced, time-serving so-called medical historians to detract from Hahnemann his historic importance for medicine, Hahnemann remains one of the four epochal figures in the history of the practice of medicine. Hippocrates, the Observer, introduced the art of clinical observation as the necessary basis for pathological diagnosis. Galen, the Disseminator, spread with powerful authority the teachings of Hippocrates over the medical world. Paracelsus, the Assailer, introduced chemical as well as physical analysis into the practice of medicine. Hahnemann, the Experimenter, discovered the symptomatic source of both pathologic and therapeutic diagnosis and thereby made the practice of medicine scientific.

In the scientific practice of medicine, we examine every patient suffering from any of the topic, plastic, trophic and toxic diseases to which man is subject, in order to obtain all the signs and symptoms of his disease, all his disease effects for pathologic and therapeutic diagnosis and prognosis. We examine by observing the pathologic and comparing it with the physiologic for diagnostic interpretation, prognostic prediction, and therapeutic application. We diagnose by classifying the pathologic condition with similar pathologic conditions. We diagnose the anatomic seat, the where, that is, the organs and the parts of the organs affected. We diagnose the physiologic process, the what, that is, the course of the inflammations, exudations, degenerations, necroses, atrophies, hypertrophies, aplasias, hyperplasias. We diagnose the etiologic factor, the how, that is, developmental, traumatic, infectious antecedents of predisposition and excitation. We diagnose the therapeutic application, the end, that is, the remedial treatment for cure and palliation, and the prophylactic treatment for hygiene and sanitation.

The treatment of patients, subject to malformations, malpositions, malnutritions, injuries, foreign bodies, traumatic and infection inflammations, new formations, is effected with medical, surgical, hygienic means, or a combination of all these in a given patient. Surgery may remove or palliate effects of anatomic excesses, defect perversions. Food, water, air, heat and cold, light and electricity, exercise and work, massage and suggestion, as well as glands to replace glands, vaccines to call out antibodies and sera to supply antibodies may remedy or palliate effects of physiologic excesses, deficiencies, perversions, may restore hygiene and establish sanitation. Medicine, in the form of medicinal substances, may remedy of palliate effects of etiologic excesses, defects, perversions, effects which are not remedies or remediable, palliated or palliable by surgery, hygienic or quasi-hygienic measures.

It is impossible to know all the antecedents causative of disease consequents. Tolle causam is easier said than done. How, then, shall we remove or palliate these effects by medical substances? Here, Hahnemann steps in to say, for the first time in all history: Remove the effects and you remove the disease, the cause of the effects. Cessat effectus cessat causa. Empiric medicine guesses, recommends, tries, hits and misses, misses and hits again. Scientific medicine does not guess. Scientific medicine, like any other scientific art, compares effects, corresponding sensations and motions. Only the mountebanks in medicine decry methods of comparison as unscientific. All that we can humanly do, and scientifically do, is to observe and classify, to compare and infer. Hahnemann says, we must apply medicinal substances on the basis of knowledge of their actual effects. Since it is impossible to know all the antecedents causative of disease consequents, we must treat the disease effects which we do know by medicinal effects which we have ascertained and know. Disease effects are removed by the application of medicines having corresponding medicinal effects. If the disease effects are removed in toto, we have a cure. If the disease effects are removed in part, we have palliation. Scientific comparison of disease effects and medicinal effects for application leads to the diagnostic inferences of scientific medicine, makes scientific medicine possible.

In 1790, Hahnemann made his celebrated experiment with china. From that time to 1839, that is, in the course of about fifty years, he experiemented with ninety-nine drugs and recorded his observations of their actions on the human body. This record, found in his "Fragmenta de Viribus Medicamentorum Positivis," "Materia Medica Pura" and "Chronic Diseases" is the largest, the most accurate and the most fertile of all investigations info medicinal action made by any single observer, before or since Hahnemann, throughout the annals of medical history.

Hahnemann was, in all essentials, a flawless experimenter. He took four drachms of china twice a day. He had paroxysms of chill and fever. In his practice as a physician he had seen similar paroxysms of chill and fever. He had cured them with china, the Peruvian bark. No longer might it be said that Peruvian bark cures paroxysms of chills and fever because Peruvian bark produces paroxysms of chills and fever. The necessity for the methodical discovery of the medicinal properties of drugs was made apparent. He who says that Hahnemann should not have experimented on himself but on dogs, or cats, or rats, or mice, has not yet entered the school of scientific logic. Disease manifests itself not merely by objective signs of sensory impression, but also by subjective symptoms of motor expression. Can the human expermenter record the subjective feelings of dogs, and cats, and rats, and mice when the dogs, and cats, and rats, and mice cannot communicate to his understanding their subjective feelings? There are no two human beings entirely the same in health and disease. Are dogs, or cats, or mice, or rats more nearly like to human beings than human beings are like to one another?

The routine experimenter, or so-called experimenter, experiments as though experiments were ends in themselves. This is the reason for the sterility of most public and private experimental stations. The experimenter experiments, but does not know why he experiments. The moral justification may be that he experiments because he is paid to experiment; but where is the scientific justification? Hahnemann had scientific justification for his experiments. That is the reason why his experiments were not sterile.

Experimentation is for one of two purposes, observation for induction, or verification of inductions. Experimentation is analysis, deduction, analytic deduction. We deduce from objects of nature, man or drug, properties in contrast with other properties. We observe by contrast. Observation is comparison, weighing, judging of contrasts. We compare for correspondence. We classify by resemblance. Classification is synthesis, induction, synthetic induction. We classify, conceive for reflection, thought, judgement. We think for expression. We formulate our propositions for verification. We verify by experimentation, by analytic deduction, the formulated propositions of science, or scientific inductions.

Hahnemann experimented for observation. He perceived in himself the symptomatic effects of Peruvian bark as similar to the symptomatic effects of intermittent fever he had removed in others with Peruvian bark. Who can say that china, taken into the healthy human body, will not produce signs, objective symptoms and feelings, subjective symptoms similar to those of intermittent fever? Hahnemann had the contrast of health without the drug and disease with the drug within himself. He was not a sterile observer. Perception led at once to conception. Hahnemann conceived the symptomatic affinity of drugs for tissues, the symptom similarity of drugs and tissues as essential for the medical treatment of medically curable diseases. If ever there was a clear scientific induction from scientific observation, it was this induction of Hahnemann's symptom similarity of drugs and tissues, which he denominated homoeopathy, and for the elucidation of which he wrote his

"Organon of Medicine" in 1810, and re-wrote it consecutively in 1819, 1824, 1829, 1833, and finally annotated and emended the 1833 edition for this sixth, his last edition, in 1842.

Was he in error? Was he premature with his conception? Hahnemann was not one of those so-called scientists who collect and catalogue their perceptual facts with no more scientific imagination than is exercised by cataloguers of libraries and collectors of taxes. Science is verified or verifiable knowledge produced by conception of percepts, induction of deducts. For scientific imagination, conceptuation from perception, not many percepts are needed. Was Pythagoras in error because, perceiving mast and sails before perceiving the hull of a ship on the horizon, he conceived that the earth is round? Was his conception premature, untrue, because everybody except Aristotle for nearly two thousand years maintained that the earth is flat, because it took nearly two thousand years before Columbus began and Magellan finished the rounding of the earth?

Hahnemann himself saw to it that there was no error in his induction. He was his own Columbus, his own Magellan. Hahnemann treated, with his own hands, his own medically curable patients and taught other medical men to treat their own medically curable patients by the method of symptom similarity he had conceived. In 1797, he used veratrum album for colic, and nux Vomica for asthma, and cured the multitudinous medically-curable patients that came to him from his sojourn in Königs-lutter to his last abiding place in Paris by this method of symptom similarity, the central method of scientific medical therapeutics. His were truly scientific verifications. Those that doubt this really do not doubt. They know not what they doubt. The verifications of Hahnemann convince those who have intellectual integrity for scientific conviction, who will not sacrifice their intellectual integrity to the idols of the day, who will repeat Hahnemann's experimental verifications of his scientific observations and inductions as they should be repeated. Any other method than to take into the healthy body four drachms of china twice a day to prove or to disprove the symptom similarity of china and intermittent fever is not a scientific experiment for the observation of Hahnemann, that there is symptom similarity between china and intermittent fever. Any other method than to administer china to patients suffering from intermittent fever to prove or to disprove the method of symptom similarity in dosage smaller than that used for exciting the healthy body into disease action similar to that of intermittent fever is not a scientific experimental verification of the induction of Hahnemann, that symptom similarity is the curative method of medically curable diseases. Those that pursue other methods have not even the frog's legs of Aristophanes to stand upon. Pasteur, perceiving that Jenner's milder cowpox prevented the appearance of the severer smallpox, conceived the prophylactic treatment of infectious diseases by milder vaccinations with the virus exciting a given infection.

How did Pasteur prove his conception? He took a number of sheep; vaccinated some of the sheep with a milder prophylactic dose of anthrax virus; then infected into all the sheep anthrax virus in larger dosage sufficient to excite anthrax; all those sheep he had vaccinated previously with the milder prophylactic anthrax virus lived without anthrax; those not vaccinated prophylactically died with anthrax. Pasteur, like the elder and greater Hahnemann, was a scientific experimented, not a would-be experimenter.

The era of scientific medical experimentation begins with Hahnemann and nobody else. Scientific to the core, Hahnemann experimented scientifically for scientific observation. Alert with intellectual power, he conceived his induction scientifically from scientific observation. Uncompromisingly scientific for experimental verification, he verified his induction scientifically for all time on his patients and made his method of symptom similarity for all time the central curative method of scientific medical therapeutics. For over a hundred years this method has been consciously and unconsciously followed by the medical profession. The results substantiate Hahnemann's contentions. There is no greater achievement than to have scientific truth, pass it on, have succeeding generations follow it and express it. Hahnemann's 'Organon of Medicine" goes out to teach symptom similarity as the experimental basis of pathologic and therapeutic diagnosis, as the *echte Heilweg* of scientific medicine.

Author's Preface to the Sixth Edition

Medicine as commonly practised (allopathy) knows no treatment except to draw from diseases the injurious materials which are assumed to be their cause. The blood of the patient is made to flow mercilessly by bleedings, leeches, cuppings, scarifications, to diminish an assumed plethora which never exists as in well women a few days before their menses, an accumulation of blood the loss of which is of no appreciable consequence, while the loss of blood with merely assumed plethora destroys life. Medicine as commonly practised seeks to evacuate the contents of the stomach and sweep the intestines clear by the materials assumed to originate diseases.

In order to give a general notion of the treatment of diseases pursued by the old school of medicine (allopathy) it may be observed that it presupposes the existence sometimes of excess of blood (plethora – which is never present), sometimes of morbid matters and acridities; hence it taps off the life's blood and exerts itself either to clear away the imaginary disease-matter or to conduct it elsewhere (by emetics, purgatives, sialogogues, diaphoretics, diuretics, drawing plasters, setons, issues, etc.), in the vain belief that the disease will thereby be weakened and materially eradicated; in place of which the patient's sufferings are thereby increased, and by such and other painful appliances the forces and nutritious juices indispensable to the curative process are abstracted from the organism. It assails the body with large doses of powerful medicines, often repeated in rapid succession for a long time, whose long-enduring, not infrequently frightful effects it knows not, and which it, purposely it would almost seem, makes unrecognisable by the commingling of several such unknown substances in one prescription, and by their long-continued employment it develops in the body new and often ineradicable medicinal diseases. Whenever it can, it employs, in order to keep in favor with its patient, [1] remedies that immediately suppress and hide the morbid symptoms by opposition (contraria contrariis) for a short time (palliatives), but that leave the cause for these symptoms (the disease itself) strengthened and aggravated. It considers affections on the exterior of the body as purely local and existing there independently, and vainly supposes that it has cured them when it has driven them away by means of external remedies, so that the internal affection is thereby compelled to break out on a nobler and more important part. When it knows not what else to do for the disease which will not yield or which grows worse, the old school of medicine undertakes to change it into something else, it knows not what, by means of an alterative, for example, by the life-undermining calornel, corrosive sublimate and other mercurial preparations in large doses.

It seems that the unhallowed principal business of the old school of medicine (allopathy) is to render incurable if not fatal the majority of diseases, those made chronic through ignorance by continually weakening and tormenting the already debilitated patient by the further addition of new destructive drug diseases.

When this pernicious practice has become a habit and one is rendered insensible to the admonitions of conscience, this becomes a very easy business indeed.

And yet for all these mischievous operations the ordinary physician of the old school can assign his reasons, which, however, rest only on foregone conclusions of his books and teachers, and on the authority of this or that distinguished physician of the old school. Even the most opposite and the most senseless modes of treatment find there their defence, their authority – let their disastrous effects speak ever so loudly against them. It is only under the old physician who has been at last gradually convinced, after many years of misdeeds, of the mischievous nature of hi so-called art, and who no longer treats even the severest diseases with anything stronger than plantain water mixed with strawberry syrup (i.e., with nothing), that the smallest number are injured and die.

This non-healing art, which for many centuries has been firmly established in full possession of the power to dispose of the life and death of patients according to its own good will and pleasure, and in that period has shortened the lives of ten times as many human beings as the most destructive wars, and rendered many millions of patients more diseased and wretched than they were originally – this allopathy, I have, in the introduction to the former editions of this book, considered more in detail. Now I shall consider only its exact opposite, the true healing art, discovered by me and now somewhat more perfected. Examples are given to prove that striking cures performed in former times were always due to remedies basically homoeopathic and found by the physician accidentally and contrary to the then prevailing methods of therapeutics.

As regards the latter (homoeopathy) it is quite otherwise. It can easily convince every reflecting person that the diseases of man are not caused by any substance, any acridity, that is to say, any disease-matter, but that they are solely spirit-like (dynamic) derangements of the spirit-like power (the vital principle) that animates the human body. Homoeopathy knows that a cure can only take place by the reaction of the vital force against the rightly chosen remedy that has been ingested, and that the cure will be certain and rapid in proportion to the strength with which the vital force still prevails in the patient. Hence homoeopathy avoids everything in the slightest degree enfeebling, [2] and as much as possible every excitation of pain, for pain also diminishes the strength, and hence it employs for the cure ONLY those medicines whose power for altering and deranging (dynamically) the health it knows accurately, and from these it selects one whose pathogenetic power (its medicinal disease) is capable of removing the natural disease in question by similarity (simila similibus), and this it administers to the patient in simple form, but in rare and minute doses so small that, without occasioning pain or weakening, they just suffice to remove the natural malady whence this result: that without weakening, injuring or torturing him in the very least, the natural disease is extinguished, and the patient, even whilst he is getting better, gains in strength and thus is cured – an apparently easy but actually troublesome and difficult business, and one requiring much thought, but which restores the patient without suffering in a short time to perfect health, – and thus it is a salutary and blessed business.

Thus homoeopathy is a perfectly simple system of medicine, remaining always fixed in its principles as in its practice, which, like the doctrine whereon it is based, if rightly apprehended will be found to be complete (and therefore serviceable). What is clearly pure in doctrine and practice should be self-evident, and all backward sliding to the pernicious routinism of the old school that is as much its antithesis as night is to day, should cease to vaunt itself with the honorable name of Homoeopathy.

Samuel Hahnemann
Paris, 1842

[1] For the same object the experienced allopath delights to invent a fixed name, by preference a Greek one, for the malady, in order to make the patient believe that he has long known this disease as an old acquaintance, and hence is the fitted person to cure it.
[2] Homoeopathy sheds not a drop of blood, administers no emetics, purgatives, laxatives or diaphoretics, drives off no external affection by external means, prescribes no hot or unknown mineral baths or medicated clysters, applies no Spanish flies or mustard plasters, no setons, no issues, excites no ptyalism, burns not with moxa or red-hot iron to the very bone, and so forth, but gives with its own hand its own preparations of simple uncompounded medicines, which it is accurately acquainted with, never subdues pain by opium, etc.

Introduction

Review of the therapeutics, allopathy and palliative treatment that have hitherto been practiced in the old school of medicine.

As long as men have existed they have been liable, individually or collectively, to diseases from physical or moral causes. In a rude state of nature but few remedial agents were required, as the simple mode of living admitted of but few diseases; with the civilization of mankind in the state, on the contrary, the occasions of diseases and the necessity for medical aid increased, in equal proportion. But ever since that time (soon after Hippocrates, therefore, for 2500 years) men have occupied themselves with the treatment of the ever increasing multiplicity of diseases, who, led astray by their vanity, sought by reasoning and guessing to excogitate the mode of furnishing this aid. Innumerable and dissimilar ideas respecting the nature of diseases and their remedies sprang from so many dissimilar brains, and the theoretical views these gave rise to the so-called systems, each of which was at variance with the rest and self-contradictory. Each of these subtle expositions at first threw the readers into stupefied amazement at the incomprehensible wisdom contained in it, and attracted to the system-monger a number of followers, who re-echoed his unnatural sophistry, to none of whom, however, was it of the slightest use in enabling them to cure better, until a new system, often diametrically opposed to the first, thrust that aside, and in its turn gained a short-lived renown. None of them, however. was in consonance with nature and experience; they were mere theoretical webs, woven by cunning intellects out of pretended consequences, which could not be made use of in practice, in the treatment at the sick-bed, on account of their excessive subtilty and repugnance to nature, and only served for empty disputations.

Simultaneously, but quite independent of all these theories, there sprung up a mode of treatment with mixtures of unknown medicinal substances for forms of disease arbitrarily set up, and directed towards some material object completely at variance with nature and experience, hence, as may be supposed, with a bad result – such is old medicine, allopathy as it is termed.

Without disparaging the services which many physicians have rendered to the sciences auxiliary to medicine, to natural philosophy and chemistry, to natural history in its various branches, and to that of man in particular, to anthropology, physiology and anatomy, etc., I shall occupy myself here with the practical part of medicine only, with the healing art itself, in order to show how it is that diseases have hitherto been so imperfectly treated. Far beneath my notice is that mechanical routine of treating precious human life according to the prescription manuals, the continual publication of which shows, alas! how frequently they are still used. I pass it by unnoticed, as a despicable practice of the lowest class of ordinary practitioners. I speak merely of the medical art as hitherto practiced, which, pluming itself on its antiquity, imagines itself to possess a scientific character.

The partisans of the old school of medicine flattered themselves that they could justly claim for it alone the title of 'rational medicine', because they alone sought for and strove to remove the cause of disease, and followed the method employed by nature in diseases.

Tolle causam! they cried incessantly. But they went no further than this empty exclamation. They only fancied that they could discover the cause of disease; they did not discover it, however, as it is not perceptible and not discoverable. For as far the greatest number of diseases are of dynamic (spiritual) origin and dynamic (spiritual) nature, their cause is therefore not perceptible to the senses; so they exerted themselves to imagine one, and from a survey of the parts of the normal, inanimate human body (anatomy), compared with the visible changes of the same internal parts in persons who had died of diseases (pathological anatomy), as also from what they could deduce from a comparison of the phenomena and functions in healthy life (physiology) with their endless alterations in the innumerable morbid states (pathology, semeiotics), to draw conclusions relative to the invisible process whereby the changes which take place in the inward being of man in diseases are affected – a dim picture of the imagination, which theoretical medicine regarded as its prima causa morbi;[1] and thus it was at one and the same time the proximate cause of the disease, and the internal essence of the disease, the disease itself – although, as sound human reason teaches us, the cause of a thing or of an event, can never be at the same time the thing or the event itself. How could they then, without deceiving themselves, consider this imperceptible internal essence as the object to be treated, and prescribe for it medicines whose curative powers were likewise generally unknown to them, and even give several such unknown medicines mixed together in what are termed prescriptions?

1. It would have been much more consonant with sound human reason and with the nature of things, had they, in order to be able to cure a disease, regarded the originating cause as the *causa morbi*, and endeavored to discover that, and thus been enabled successfully to employ the mode of treatment which had shown itself useful in maladies having the same exciting cause, in those also of a similar origin, as, for example, the same mercury is efficacious in an ulcer of the glans after impure coitus, as in all previous venereal chancres – if, I say, they had discovered the exciting cause of all other (non-venereal) chronic diseases to be an infection at one period or another with the itch miasm (psora), and had found for all these a common method of treatment, regard being had for the peculiarities of each individual case, whereby all and each of these chronic diseases might have been cured, then might they with justice have boasted that in the treatment of chronic diseases they had in view the only available and useful *causa morborum chronicorum* (*non venereorum*), and with this as a basis they might have treated such diseases with the best results. But during these many centuries they were unable to cure the millions of chronic diseases, because they knew not their origin in the psoric miasm (which was first discovered and afterwards provided with a suitable plan of treatment by homoeopathy), and yet they vaunted that they alone kept in view the prima causa of these diseases in their treatment, and that they alone treated rationally, although they had not the slightest conception of the only useful knowledge of their psoric origin and consequently they bungled the treatment of all chronic diseases!

But this sublime problem, the discovery, namely, a priori, of an internal invisible cause of disease, resolved itself, at least with the more astute physicians of the old school, into a search, under the guidance of the symptoms it is true, for what might be supposed to be the probable general character of the case of disease before them;[2] whether it was spasm, or debility, or paralysis, or fever, or inflammation, or induration, or obstruction of this or that part, or excess of blood (plethora), deficiency or excess of oxygen, carbon, hydrogen or nitrogen in the juices, exaltation or depression of the functions of the arterial, venous or capillary system, change in the relative proportion of the factors of sensibility, irritability or reproduction., – conjectures that have been dignified by the followers of the old school with the title of causal indication, and considered to be the only possible rationality in medicine; but which were assumptions, too fallacious and hypothetical to prove of any practical utility – incapable, even had they been well grounded, of indicating the most appropriate remedy for a case of disease; flattering indeed, to the vanity of the learned theorist, but usually leading astray when used as guides to practice, and wherein there was evidenced more of ostentation than of an earnest search for the curative indication.

2. Every physician who treats disease according to such general character however he may affect to claim the name of homoeopathist, is and ever will remain in fact a generalising allopath, for without the most minute individualisation, homoeopathy is not conceivable.

And how often has it happened that, for example, spasm or paralysis seemed to be in one part of the organism, while in another part inflammation was apparently present!

Or, on the other hand, whence are the certain remedies for each of these pretended general characters to be derived? Those that would certainly be of benefit could be none other than the specific medicines, that is, those whose action is homogeneous[3] to the morbid irritation; whose employment, however, is denounced and forbidden[4] by the old school as highly injurious, because observation has shown that in consequence of the receptivity for homogeneous irritation being so highly increased in diseases, such medicines in the usual large doses are dangerous to life. The old school never dreamt of smaller, and of extremely small doses. Accordingly no attempt was made to cure, in the direct (the most natural) way, by means of homogeneous, specific medicines; nor could it be done, as the effects of most of medicines were, and continued to remain, unknown, and even had they been known it would have been impossible to hit on the right medicine with such generalizing views as were entertained.

3. Now termed Homoeopathic.

4. "Where experience showed the curative power of homoeopathically acting remedies, whose mode of action could not be explained, the difficulty was avoided by calling them specific, and further investigation was stifled by this actually unmeaning word. The homogeneous excitant remedies, the specific (homoeopathic), medicines, however, had long previously been prohibited as of very injurious influence". – Rau, On the Value of the homoeopathic Method of Treatment, Heidelberg, 1824, pp. 101, 102.

However, perceiving that it was more consistent with reason to seek for another path, a straight one if possible, rather than to take circuitous courses, the old school of medicine believed it might cure diseases in a direct manner by the removal of the (imaginary) material cause of disease – for to physicians of the ordinary school, while investigating and forming a judgment upon a disease, and not less while seeking for the curative indication, it was next to impossible to divest themselves of these materialistic ideas, and to regard the nature of the spiritual-corporeal organism as such a highly potentialized entity, that its sensational and functional vital changes, which are called diseases, must be produced and effected chiefly, if not solely, by dynamic (spiritual) influences, and could not be effected in any other way.

The old school regarded all those matters which were altered by the disease, those abnormal matters that occurred in congestions, as well as those that were excreted, as disease-producers, or at least on account of their supposed reacting power, as disease maintainers, and this latter notion prevails to this day.

Hence they dreamed of effecting causal cures by endeavoring to remove these imaginary and presumed material causes of the disease. Hence their assiduous evacuation of the bile by vomiting in bilious fevers;5 their emetics in cases of so-called stomach derangenments;6 their diligent purging away of the mucus, the lumbrici and the ascarides in children who are pale-faced and who suffer from ravenous appetite, bellyache, and enlarged abdomen7; their venesections in cases of haemorrhage;8and more especially all their varieties of blood-lettings,9 their main remedy in inflammations, which they now, following the example of a well-known bloodthirsty Parisian physician (as a flock of sheep follow the bell-wether even into the butcher's slaughter-house), imagine to encounter in almost every morbidly affected part of the body, and feel themselves, bound to remove by the application of often a fatal number of leeches. They believe that by so doing they obey the true casual indications, and treat disease in a rational manner. The adherents of the old school, moreover, believe that by putting a ligature on polypi, by cutting out, or artificially exciting suppuration by means of local irritants in indolent glandular swellings, by enucleating encysted tumors (steatoma and meliceria) by their operations for aneurysm and lacrymal and anal fistula, by removing with the knife scirrhous tumors of the breast, by amputating a limb affected with necrosis, etc., they cure the patient radically, and that their treatment is directed against the cause of the disease; and they also think, when they employ their repellent remedies, dry up old running ulcers in the legs with astringent applications of oxide of lead copper or zinc (aided always by the simultaneous administration of purgatives, which merely debilitate, but have no effect on the fundamental dyscrasia), cauterize chancres, destroy condylomata locally, drive off itch from the skin with ointments of sulphur, oxide of lead, mercury or zinc, suppress ophthalmiae with solutions of lead or zinc, and drive away tearing pains from the limbs by means of opodeldoc, hartshorn liniment or fumigations with cinnabar or amber; in every case they think they have removed the affection, conquered the disease, and pursued a rational treatment directed towards the cause. But what is the result! The metastatic affections that sooner or later, but inevitably appear, caused by this mode of treatment (but which they pretend are entirely new diseases), which are always worse than the original malady, sufficiently prove their error, and might and should open their eyes to the deeper-seated, immaterial nature of the disease, and its dynamic (spirit-like) origin, which can only be removed by dynamic means.

5. The estimable Hofrath Dr. Fau (loc. cit., p.176) at a time when not properly conversant with homoeopathy, by firmly convince the dynamic cause of these fevers, cured them without employing an evacuation remedy, by means of one or two small doses of homoeopathic remedies, two very remarkable cases of which he relates in his book.

6. In a case of sudden derangement of the stomach, with constant disgusting eructations with the taste of the vitiated food, generally accompanied by depression of spirits, cold hands and feet, etc., the ordinary physician has hitherto been in the habit of attacking only the degenerated contents of the stomach; a powerful emetic should clean it out completely. This object was generally attained by tartar emetic, with or without ipecacuanha. Does the patient, however, immediately after this become well, brisk and cheerful? Oh, no! Such a derangement of the stomach is usually of dynamic origin, caused by mental disturbance (grief, fright, vexation), a chill, over-exertion of the mund or body immediately after eating, often after even a moderate meal. Those two remedies are not suitable for removing this dynamic derangement, and just as little is the revolutionary vomiting they produce. Moreover, tartar emetic and ipecacuanha, from their other peculiar pathogenetic powers, prove of further injury to the patient's health, and derange the biliary secretion; so that if the patient be not very robust, he must feel ill for several days from the effects of this pretended causal treatment, notwithstanding all this violent expulsion of the whole contents of the stomach. If the patient, however, in place of taking such violent and always (a) hurtful evacuant drugs, smell only a single time at a globule the size of a mustard seed, moistened with highly diluted pulsatillajuice, whereby the derangement of his health in general and of his stomach in particular will certainly be removed, in two hours he is quite well; and if the eructation recur once more, it consists of tasteless and inodorous air; the contents of the stomach cease to be vitiated, and at the next meal he has regained his full usual appetite; he is quite well and lively. This is true causal medication; the former is only an imaginary one and has an injurious effect on the patient.

Even a stomach overloaded with indigestible food never requires a medicinal emetic. In such a case nature is competent to rid herself of the excess in the best way through the oesophagus, by means of nausea, sickness and spontaneous vomiting, assisted, it may be, by mechanical irritation of the palate and fauces, and by this means the accessory medicinal effects of the emetic drugs are avoided; a small quantity of coffee expedites the passage downwards of what remains in the stomach.

But if, after excessive overloading of the stomach, the irritability of the stomach is not sufficient to promote spontaneous vomiting, or is lost altogether, so that the tendency thereto is extinguished, while there are at the same time great pains in the epigastrium, in such a paralyzed state of the stomach, an emetic medicine would only have the effect of producing a dangerous or fatal inflammation of the intestines; where a small quantity of strong infusion of coffee, frequently administered, would dynamically exalt the sunken irritability of the stomach, and put it in a condition to expel its contents, be they ever so great, either upwards or downwards. So here also the pretended causal treatment is out of place.

Even the acrid gastric acid, to eructations of which patients with chronic diseases are not infrequently subject, may be today violently evacuated by means of an emetic, with great suffering, and yet all in vain, for tomorrow or some days later it is replaced by similar acrid gastric acid, and then usually in larger quantities; whereas it goes away by itself when its dynamic cause is removed by a very small dose of a high dilution of sulphuric acid, or still better, if it is of frequent recurrence, by the employment of minutest doses of antipsoric remedies corresponding in similarity to the rest of the symptoms also. And of a similar character are many of the pretended causal cures of the old-school physicians, whose main effort it is, by means of tedious operations, troublesome to themselves and injurious to their patients, to clear away the material product of the dynamic derangement; whereas if they perceived the dynamic source of the affection, and annihilated it and its products homoeopathically, they would thereby effect a rational cure.

7. Conditions dependent solely on a psoric taint, and easily curable by mild (dynamic) antipsoric remedies without emetics or purgatives.

8. Notwithstanding that almost all morbid haemorrhages depend on a dynamic derangement of the vital force (state of health), yet the old-school physicians consider their cause to be excess of blood, and cannot refrain from bleeding in order to draw off the supposed superabundance of this vital fluid; the palpable evil consequences of which procedure, however, such as prostration of the strength, and the tendency or actual transition, to the typhoid state they ascribe to the malignancy of the disease, which they are then often unable to overcome – in fine, they imagine, even when the patient does not recover, that their treatment has been in conformity with their axiom, *causam tolle*, and that, according to their mode of speaking, they have done everything in their power for the patient, let the result be what it may.

9. Although there probably never was a drop of blood too much in the living human body, yet the old-school practitioners consider an imaginary excess of blood as the main material cause of all haemorrhages and inflammations, which they must remove and drain off by venesections, cupping and leeches. This they hold to be a rational mode of treatment, causal medication. In general inflammatory fevers, in acute pleurisy, they even regard the coagulable lymph in the blood – the buffy coat, as it is termed – as the *materia peccans*, which they endeavor to get rid of, if possible, by repeated venesections, notwithstanding that this coat often becomes more consistent and thicker at every repetition of the bloodletting. They thus often bleed the patient nearly to death, when the inflammatory fever will not subside, in order to remove this buffy coat or the imaginary plethora, without suspecting that the inflammatory blood is only the product of the acute fever, of the morbid, immaterial (dynamic) inflammatory irritation, and that the latter is the sole cause of the great disturbance in the vascular system, and may be removed by the smallest dose of a homogeneous (homoeopathic) medicine, as, for instance, by a small globule of the decillion-fold dilution of aconite juice, with abstinence from vegetable acids, so that the most violent pleuritic fever, with all its alarming concomitants, is changed into health and cured, without the least abstraction of blood and without any antiphlogistic remedy, in a few – at the most in twenty-four – hours (a small quantity of blood drawn from a vein by the way of experiment then shows no traces of buffy coat); whereas another patient similarly affected, and treated on the rational principles of the old school, if, after repeated bleedings, with great difficulty and unspeakable sufferings he escape for the nonce with life, he often has still many months to drag through before he can support his emaciated body on his legs, if in the mean time (as often happens from such maltreatment) he be not carried off by typhoid fever, leucophlegmasia or pulmonary phthisis.

Anyone who has felt the tranquil pulse of a man an hour before the occurrence of the rigor that always precedes an attack of acute pleurisy, will not be able to restrain his amazement if told two hours later, after the hot stage has commenced, that the enormous plethora present urgently requires repeated venesections, and will naturally inquire by what magic power could the pounds of blood that must now be drawn off have been conjured into the blood-vessels of this man within these two hours, which but two hours previously he had felt beating in such a tranquil manner. Not a single drachm more of blood can now be circulating in those vessels than existed when he was in good health, not yet two hours ago!

Accordingly the allopathic physician with his venesections draws from the patient laboring under acute fever no oppressive superabundance of blood, as that cannot possibly be present; he only robs him of what is indispensable to life and recovery, the normal quantity of blood and consequently of strength – a great loss which no physician's power can replaced – and yet he vainly imagines that he has conducted the treatment in conformity to his (misunderstood) axiom, *causam tolle*; whereas it is impossible that the *causa morbi* in this case can be an excess of blood, which is not present; but the sole true *causa morbi* was a morbid, dynamical, inflammatory irritation of the circulatory system, as is proved by the rapid and permanent cure of this and every similar case of general inflammatory fever by one or two inconceivably minute doses of aconite juice, which removes such an irritation homoeopathically.

The old school errs equally in the treatment of local inflammations with its topical bloodlettings, more especially with the quantities of leeches which are now applied according to the maniacal principles of Broussai's. The palliative amelioration that at first ensues from the treatment is far from being crowned by a rapid and perfect cure; on the contrary, the weak and ailing state of the parts thus treated (frequently also of the whole body), which always remains, sufficiently shows the error that is committed in attributing the local inflammation to a local plethora, and how sad are the consequences of such abstractions of blood; whereas this purely dynamic, apparently local, inflammatory irritation, can be rapidly and permanently removed by an equally small dose of aconite, or, according to circumstances, of belladonna, and the whole disease annihilated and cured, without such unjustifiable shedding of blood.

A favorite idea of the ordinary school of medicine, until recent (would that I could not say the most recent) times, was that of morbific matters (and acridities) in diseases, excessively subtle though they might be thought to be, which must be expelled from the blood-vessels and lymphathics, through the exhalents, skin, urinary apparatus or salivary glands, through the tracheal and bronchial glands in the form of expectoration, from the stomach and bowels by vomiting and purging, in order that the body might be freed from the material cause that produced the disease, and a radical causal treatment be thus carried out.

By cutting holes in the diseased body, which were converted into chronic ulcers kept up for years by the introduction of foreign substances (issues, setons), they sought to draw off the *materia peccans* from the (always only dynamically) diseased body, just as one lets a dirty fluid run out of a barrel through the taphole. By means also of perpetual fly-blisters and the application of mezereum, they thought to draw away the bad humors and to cleanse the diseased body from all morbific matters – but they only weakened it, so as generally to render it incurable, by all these senseless unnatural processes.

I admit that it was more convenient for the weakness of humanity to assume that, in the diseases they were called on to cure, there existed some morbific material of which the mind might form a conception (more particularly as the patients readily lent themselves to such a notion), because in that case the practitioner had nothing further to care about than to procure a good supply of remedies for purifying the blood and humors, exciting diuresis and diaphoresis, promoting expectoration, and scouring out the stomach and bowels. Hence, in all the works on Materia Medica, from Dioscorides down to the latest books on this subject, there is almost nothing said about the special peculiar action of individual medicines; but, besides on account of their supposed utility in various nosological names of diseases, it is merely stated whether they are diuretic, diaphoretic, expectorant or emmenagogue, and more particularly whether they produce evacuation of the stomach and bowels upwards or downwards; because all the aspirations and efforts of the practitioner have ever been chiefly directed to cause the expulsion of a material morbific matter, and of sundry (fictitious) acridities, which it was imagined were the cause of diseases.

These were, however, all idle dreams, unfounded assumptions and hypotheses, cunningly devised for the convenience of therapeutics, as it was expected the easiest way of performing a cure would be to remove the material morbific matters *(si modo essent!)*.

But the essential nature of diseases and their cure will not adapt themselves to such fantasies, nor to the convenience of medical men; to humor such stupid baseless hypotheses diseases will not cease to be (spiritual) dynamic derangements of our spirit-like vital principle in sensations and functions, that is to say, immaterial derangements of our state of health.

The causes of our maladies cannot be material, since the least foreign material substance, however mild it may appear to us, if introduced into our blood-vessels, is promptly ejected by the vital force, as though it were a poison; or when this does not happen, death ensues. If even the minutes splinter penetrates a sensitive part of our organism, the vital principle everywhere present in our body never rests until it is removed by pain, fever, suppuration or gangrene. And can it be supposed that in a case of cutaneous disease of twenty years standing, for instance, this indefatigably active vital principle will quietly endure the presence of such an injurious foreign, material exanthematous substance, such as a herpetic, a scrofulous, a gouty acridity, etc., in the fluids of the body? Did any nosologist ever see with corporeal eyes such a morbific matter, to warrant him in speaking so confidently about it, and in founding a system of medical treatment upon it? Has any one ever succeeded in displaying to view the matter of gout or the poison of scrofula?

10. Life was endangered by injecting a little pure water into a vein. (Vide Mullen, quoted by Birch in the History of the Royal Society.)

Atmospheric air injected into the blood-vessels caused death. (Vide J. M. Voigt, Magazin fur den neuesten Zustand der Naturkunde, i, iii, p. 25.)

Even the mildest fluids introduced into the veins endangered life. (Vide Autenreith, Physiologie, ii, Ã› 784.)

Even when the application of a material substance to the skin, or to a wound, has propagated diseases by infection, who can prove (what is so often maintained in works on pathology) that some material portion of this substance has penetrated into our fluids or been absorbed?11 The most careful and prompt washing of the genitals does not protect the system from infection with the venereal chancrous disease. The slightest breath of air emanating from the body of a person affected with smallpox will suffice to produce this horrible disease in a healthy child.

11. A girl in Glasgow, eight years of age, having been bit by a mad dog, the surgeon immediately cut the piece clean out, and yet thirty-six days afterwards she was seized with hydrophobia, which killed her in two days. (Med. Comment. of Edinb., Dec. 2, vol. ii, 1793.)

What ponderable quantity of material substance could have been absorbed into the fluids, in order to develop, in the first of these instances, a tedious dyscrasia (syphilis), which when uncured is only extinguished with the remotest period of life, with death; in the last, a disease (smallpox) accompanied by almost general suppuration, and often rapidly fatal? In these and all similar cases is it possible to entertain the idea of a material morbific matter being introduced into the blood? A letter written in the sick-room at a great distance has often communicated the same contagious disease to the person who read it. In this instance, can the notion of a material morbific matter having penetrated into the fluids be admitted? But what need is there of all such proofs? How often has it happened that an irritating word has brought on a dangerous bilious fever; a superstitious prediction of death has caused the fatal catastrophe at the very time announced; the abrupt communication of sad or excessively joyful news has occasioned sudden death? In these cases, where is the material morbific principle that entered in substance into the body, there to produce and keep up the disease, and without the material expulsion and ejection of which a radical cure were impossible?

12. In order to account for the large quantity of putrid exerementitious matter and foetid discharge often met with in diseases, and to be able to represent them as the material substance that excites and keeps up disease – although, when infection occurs, nothing perceptible in the shape of miasm, nothing material, could have penetrated into the body – recourse was had to the hypothesis, that the matter of infection, be it ever so minute, acts in the body like a ferment, bringing the fluids into a like state of corruption, and thus changing them into a similar morbific ferment which constantly increases with the disease and keeps it up. But by what all-potent and all-wise purifying draughts will you purge and cleanse the human fluids from this ever reproductive ferment, from this mass of imaginary morbific matter, and that so perfectly, that there shall not remain a particle of such morbific ferment, which, according to this hypothesis, must ever again, as at first, transform and corrupt the fluids to new morbific matter? Were that so it would evidently be impossible to cure these diseases in your way! – See how all hypotheses, be they ever so ingeniously framed, lead to the most palpable absurdities when they are not founded on truth! – The most deeply rooted syphilis may be cured, after the removal of the psora with which it is often complicated, by one or two small doses of the decillionfiold diluted and potentised solution of mercury, whereby the general syphilitic taint of the fluids is forever (dynamically) annihilated and removed.

The champions of this clumsy doctrine of morbific matters ought to be ashamed that they have so inconsiderately overlooked and failed to appreciate the spiritual nature of life, and the spiritual dynamic power of the exciting causes of diseases, and that they have thereby degraded themselves into mere scavenger-doctors, who, in their efforts to expel from the diseased body morbific matters that never existed, in place of curing, destroy life.

Are, then, the foul, often disgusting excretions which occur in diseases the actual matter that produces and keeps them up? Are they not rather always excretory products of the disease itself, that is, of the life which is only dynamically deranged and disordered?

13. Were this the case, the most inveterate coryza should be certainly and rapidly cured by merely blowing and wiping the nose carefully.

With such false and materialistic views concerning the origin and essential nature of diseases, it was certainly not to be wondered at that in all ages the main endeavor of the most obscure, as well as of the most distinguished practitioners, and even of the inventors of the sublimest medical systems, was always only to separate and expel an imaginary morbific matter, and the indication most frequently laid down was to break up and put in motion this morbific matter, to effect its expulsion by salivation, expectoration, diaphoresis and diuresis, to purify the blood from (acridities and impurities) morbific matters, which never existed, by means of the intelligence of sundry obedient decoctions of root and plants; to draw off mechanically the imaginary matter of disease by setons, by issues, by portions of the skin kept open and discharging by means of perpetual blisters or mezereum bark, but chiefly to expel and purge away the *materia peccans*, or the injurious matters as they were termed, through the intestines, by means of laxative and purgative medicines, which, in order to give them a more profound meaning and a more prepossessing appearance, were fondly denominated dissolvents and mild aperients – all so many arrangements for the expulsion of inimical morbific matters, which never could be, and never were instrumental in the production and maintenance of the diseases of the human organism, animated as it is by a spiritual principle – of diseases which never were anything else than spiritual dynamic derangements of the life altered in its sensations and functions.

Let it be granted now, what cannot be doubted, that no diseases – if they do not result from the introduction of perfectly indigestible or otherwise injurious substances into the stomach, or into other orifices or cavities of the body, or from foreign bodies penetrating. the skin, etc. – that no disease, in a word, is caused by any material substance, but that every one is only and always a peculiar, virtual, dynamic derangement of the health; how injudicious, in that case, must not a method of treatment directed towards the expulsion of that imaginary material substance appear to every rational man, since no good, but only monstrous harm, can result from its employment in the principal diseases of mankind, namely, those of a chronic character!

14. There is a semblance of necessity in the expulsion by purgatives of worms, in so-called vermicular diseases. But even this semblance is false. A few lumbric; may be found in some children; in many there exist ascarides. But the presence of these is always dependent on a general taint of the constitution (the psoric), joined to an unhealthy mode of living. Let the latter be improved, and the former cured homoeopathically, which is most easily effected at this age, and none of the worms remain, and children cured in this manner are never troubled with them more; whereas after mere purgatives, even when combined with cina seeds, they soon reappear in quantities.

"But the tapeworm", methinks I hear some one exclaim, "every effort should be made to expel that monster, which was created for the torment of mankind".

Yes, sometimes it is expelled; but at the cost of what after-sufferings, and with what danger to life! I should not like to have on my conscience the deaths of so many hundreds of human beings as have fallen sacrifices to the horribly violent purgatives, directed against the tapeworm, or the many years of indisposition of those who have escaped being purged to death. And how often does it happen that after all this health-and-life-destroying purgative treatment, frequently continued for several years, the animal is not expelled, or if so, that it is again produced!

What if there is not the slightest necessity for all these violent, cruel, and dangerous efforts to expel and kill the worm. The various species of tapeworm are only found along with the psoric taint, and always disappear when that is cured. But even before the cure is accomplished, they live – the patient enjoying tolerable health the while – not exactly in the intestines, but in the residue of the food, the excrement of the bowels, as in their proper element, quite quietly, and without causing the least disturbance, and find in the excrement what suffices for their nourishment; they then do not touch the walls of the intestine, and are perfectly harmless. But if the patient happens to be affected with an acute disease of any kind, then the contents of the bowels become intolerable to the animal; it twists about, comes in contact with, and irritates the sensitive walls of the intestines, causing a peculiar kind of spasmodic colic, which increases materially the sufferings of the patient. (So also the foetus in the womb becomes restless, turns about and kicks, only when the mother is ill; but when she is well; it swims quiet in its proper fluid without causing her any suffering.)

It is worthy of remark, that the morbid symptoms of patients suffering from tapeworm are generally of such a kind, that they are rapidly relieved (homoeopathically) by the smallest dose of tincture of male-fern root; [Filix Mas-Aspidium] so that the ill-health of the patient, which causes this parasitic animal to be restless, is thereby for the time removed; the tapeworm then feels at ease, and lives on quietly in the excrement of the bowels, without particularly distressing the patient or his intestines, until the antipsoric treatment is so far advanced that the worm, after the eradication of the psora, finds the contents of the bowels no longer suitable for its support, and therefore spontaneously disappears, for ever from the now cured patient, without the least purgative medicine.

In short, the degenerated substances and impurities that appear in diseases are, undeniably, nothing more than products of the disease of the abnormally deranged organism, which are expelled by the latter, often violently enough – often much too violently – without requiring the aid of the evacuating art, and fresh products are always developed as long as it labors under that disease. These matters the true physician regards as actual symptoms of the disease, and they aid him to discover the nature of the disease, and to form an accurate portrait of it, so as to enable him to cure it with a similar medicinal morbific agent.

But the more modern adherents of the old school do not wish it to be supposed, that in their treatment they aim at the expulsion of material morbific substances. They allege that their multifarious evacuant processes are a mode of treatment by derivation, wherein they follow the example of nature which, in her efforts to assist the diseased organism, resolves fever by perspiration and diuresis pleurisy by epistaxis, sweat and mucous expectoration – other diseases by vomiting, diarrhaea and bleeding from the anus, articular pains by suppurating ulcers on the legs, cynanche tonsillaris by salivation, etc., or removes them by metastases and abscesses which she develops in parts at a distance from the seat of the disease.

Hence they thought the best thing to do was to imitate nature, by also going to work in the treatment of most diseases in a circuitous manner like the diseased vital force when left to itself and thus in an indirect manner,15 by means of stronger heterogeneous irritants applied to organs remote from the seat of disease, and totally dissimilar to the affected tissues, they produce evacuations, and generally kept them up, in order to draw, as it were, the disease thither.

15. In place of extinguishing the disease rapidly, without exhaustion of the strength and without going about the bush, with homogeneous, dynamic medicinal agents acting directly on the diseased points of the organism, as homoeopathy does.

This derivation, as it is called, was and continues to be one of the principal modes of treatment of the old school of medicine.

In this imitation of the self-aiding operation of nature, as some call it, they endeavored to excite, by force, new symptoms in the tissues that are least diseased and best able to bear the medicinal disease, which should draw away the primary disease under the semblance of crises and under the form of excretions, in order to admit of a gradual lysis by the curative powers of nature.

16. Just as if anything immaterial could be drawn away! So that here too was the notion of a substance and a morbific matter, excessively subtle though it might be supposed to be!

17. It is only the slighter and acute diseases that tend, when the natural period of their course has expired, to terminate quietly in resolution, as it is called, with or without the employment of not very aggressive allopathic remedies; the vital force, having regained its powers, then gradually substitutes the normal condition for the derangement of the health that has now ceased to exist. But in severe acute and in chronic diseases which constitute by far the greater portion of all human ailments, crude nature and the old school are equally powerless; in these, neither the vital force, with its self-aiding faculty, nor allopathy in imitation of it, can affect a lysis, but at the most a mere temporary truce, during which the enemy fortifies himself, in order, sooner or later, to recommence the attack with still greater violence.

This they accomplished by means of diaphoretic and diuretic remedies, bloodlettings, setons and issues, but chiefly by irritant drugs to cause evacuation of the alimentary canal, sometimes upwards by means of emetics, sometimes (and this was the favorite plan) downwards by means of purgatives, which were termed aperient and dissolvent18 remedies.

18. An expression which likewise betrays that they imagined and presupposed a morbific substance, which had to be dissolved and expelled.

To assist this derivative method they employed the allied treatment by counter-irritants; woolen garments to the bare skin, foot-baths, nauseants, inflicting on the stomach and bowels the pangs of hunger (the hunger-treatment), substances to cause pain, inflammation, and suppuration in near or distant parts as the application of horseradish, mustard plasters, cantharides, blisters, mezereum setons, issues, tartar-emetic ointment, moxa, actual cautery, acupuncture, etc.; here also following the example of crude unassisted nature, which endeavors to free herself from the dynamic disease (in the case of a chronic disease, unavailingly) by exciting pain in distant parts of the body, by metastases and abscesses, by eruptions and suppurating ulcers.

It was evidently no rational principle, but merely imitation, with the view of making practice easy that seduced the old school into those unhelpful and injurious indirect modes of treatment, the derivative as well as the counter-irritant; that led them to this inefficacious, debilitating and hurtful practice of apparently ameliorating diseases for a short time, or removing them in such a manner that another and a worse disease was roused up to occupy the place of the first. Such a destructive plan cannot certainly be termed curing.

They merely followed the example of crude instinctive nature in her efforts, which are barely19 successful even in the slighter cases of acute disease; they merely imitated the unreasoning life-preserving power when left to itself in diseases, which entirely dependent as it is upon the organic laws of the body, is only capable of acting in conformity with these laws and is not guided by reason and reflection – they copied nature, which cannot, like an intelligent surgeon, bring together the gaping lips of a wound and by their union effect a cure; which knows not how to straighten and adjust the broken ends of a bone lying far apart and exuding much (often an excess of) new osseous matter; which cannot put a ligature on a wounded artery, but in its energy causes the patient to bleed to death; which does not understand how to replace a dislocated shoulder, but by the swelling it occasions round about it soon presents an obstacle to reduction; which in order to remove a foreign body from the cornea, destroys the whole eye by suppuration; which, with all its efforts can only liberate a strangulated hernia by gangrene of the bowel and death; and which, by the metaschematisms it produces in dynamic diseases, often renders them much worse than they were originally. But more, this irrational vital force receives into our body without hesitation, the greatest plagues of our terrestrial existence, the spark that kindles the countless diseases beneath which tortured mankind has groaned for hundreds and thousands of year, the chronic miasmspsora, syphilis, sycosis – not one of which can it diminish in the slightest degree far less expel single-handed from the organism; on the contrary, it allows them to rankle therein until often after a long life of misery, death at last closes the eyes of the sufferer.

19. In the ordinary school of medicine, the efforts made by nature for the relief of the organism in diseases where no medicine was given, were regarded as models of treatment worthy of imitation. But this was a great error. The pitiable and highly imperfect efforts of the vital force to relieve itself in acute diseases is a spectacle that should excite our compassion, and command the aid of all the powers of our rational mind, to terminate the self-inflicted torture by a real cure. If nature is unable to cure homoeopathically a disease already existing in the organism, by the production of another fresh malady similar to it (¤ 43-46), which very rarely lies in her power (¤ 50), and if to the organism alone is left the task of overcoming, by its own forces without external aid, a disease newly contracted (in cases of chronic miasms its power of resistance is quite inefficacious), we then witness nought but painful, often dangerous, efforts of nature to save the individual at whatever cost, which often terminate in extinction of the earthly existence, in death.

Little as we mortals know of the operations that take place in the interior economy in health – which must be hidden from us as certainly as they are patent to the eye of the all-seeing Creator and Preserver of his creatures – just as little can we perceive the operations that go on in the interior in disturbed conditions of life, in diseases. The internal operations in diseases are manifested only by the visible changes, the sufferings and the symptoms, whereby alone our life betrays the inward disturbance; so that in no given case can we ascertain which of the morbid symptoms are caused by the primary action of the morbific agent, which by the reaction of the vital force for its own relief. Both are inextricably mixed up together before our eyes, and only present to us an outwardly reflected picture of the entire internal malady, for the fruitless efforts of unassisted vitality to terminate the sufferings are themselves sufferings of the whole organism. Hence, even in those evacuations termed crises, which nature generally produces at the termination of diseases which run a rapid course, there is frequently more of suffering than of efficacious relief.

What the vital force does in these so-called crises, and how it does it, remains a mystery to us, like all the internal operations of the organic vital economy. One thing, however, is certain: that in all these efforts more or less of the affected parts are sacrificed and destroyed in order to save the rest. These self-aiding operations of the vital force for the removal of an acute disease, performed only in obedience to the laws of organic life and not guided by the reflection of an intellect, are mostly but a species of allopathy; in order to relieve the primarily affected organ by a crisis, an increased, often violent, activity is excited in the excretory organs, to draw away the disease from the former to the latter; there ensue vomitings, purgings, diuresis, diaphoresis, abscesses, etc., in order, by this irritation of distant parts, to effect a sort of derivation from the primarily diseased part, and the dynamically affected nervous power seems to unload itself in the material product.

It is only by the destruction and sacrifice of a portion of the organism itself that unaided nature can save the patient in acute diseases, and, if death do not ensue, restore, though only slowly and imperfectly, the harmony of life – health.

The great weakness of the parts which had been exposed to the disease, and even of the whole body, the emaciation, etc., remaining after spontaneous cures, are convincing proofs of this.

In short, the whole operation of the self-aiding power of the organism when attacked by diseases displays to the observer nothing but suffering – nothing that he could or ought to imitate if he wishes to cure disease in a truly artistic manner.

In such an important affair as that of healing, which demands so much intelligence, reflection and judgment, how could the old school, which arrogates to itself the title of rational, choose as its best instructor, as its guide to be blindly followed, the unintelligent vital force, inconsiderately copy its indirect and revolutionary operations in diseases, imagining these to be the non plus ultra, the best conceivable, when that greatest gift of God, reflective reason and unfettered judgment, was given us to enable us infinitely to surpass it in salutary help to suffering humanity?

When the old school practitioners, thoughtlessly imitating the crude, senseless, automatic vital energy with their counter-irritant and derivative methods of treatment – by far their most usual plans – attack innocent parts and organs of the body, either inflicting on them excruciating pains, or as is most frequently done, compelling them to perform evacuations whereby strength and fluids are wasted, their object is to direct the morbid vital action in the primarily affected parts away to those artificially attacked, and thus to effect the cure of the natural disease indirectly, by the production of a disease much greater in intensity and of quite a different kind, in the healthy parts of the body, consequently by a circuitous way, at the cost of much loss of strength, and usually of great suffering to the patient.

20. Daily experience shows the sad effects of this manoeuvre in chronic diseases. Anything but a cure is effected. Who would ever call that a victory if, in place of attacking the enemy in front in a hand-to-hand fight, and by his destruction terminating at once his hostile assaults, we should, in a cowardly manner and behind his back, lay an embargo on everything, cut off his supplies, burn down everything for a great way round him? By so doing we would at length deprive him of all courage to resist, but our object is not gained, the enemy is far from being destroyed, – he is still there, and when he can again procure provisions and supplies, he once more rears his head, more exasperated than before – the enemy, I repeat, is far from being destroyed, but the poor innocent country is so completely ruined that it will be long before it can recover itself. In like manner acts allopathy in chronic diseases, when, by its indirect attacks on innocent parts at a distance from the seat of the disease, instead of effecting a cure, it destroys the organism. Such is the result of its hurtful operations!

The disease, if it be acute, and consequently naturally of but short duration, may certainly disappear, even during these heterogeneous attacks on distant and dissimilar parts – but it is not cured. There is nothing that can merit the honorable name of cure in this revolutionary treatment, which has no direct, immediate, pathological relation to the tissues primarily affected. Often indeed, without these serious attacks on the rest of the organism, would the acute disease have ceased of itself, sooner most likely, with fewer subsequent sufferings and less sacrifice of strength. But neither the mode of operation of the crude natural forces, nor the allopathic copy of that, can for a moment be compared to the dynamic (homoeopathic) treatment, which sustains the strength, while it extinguishes the disease in a direct and rapid manner.

In far the greatest number of cases of disease, however – I mean those of a chronic nature – these perturbing, debilitating, indirect modes of treatment of the old school are scarcely ever of the slightest use. They suspend for a few days only, some troublesome symptom or other, which, however, returns when the system has become accustomed to the distant irritation, and the disease recurs worse than before, because by the antagonistic pains and the injudicious evacuations the vital powers have been depressed.

21. What good results have ever ensued from those foetid artificial ulcers, so much in vogue, called issues? If even during the first week or two, whilst they still cause pain, they appear somewhat to check by antagonism a chronic disease, yer by and by, when the body has become accustomed to the pain, they have no other effect than that of weakening the patient and giving still greater scope to the chronic affection. Or does anyone imagine, in this nineteenth century, that they serve as an outlet for the escape of the *materia peccans*? It almost appears as if this were the case!

Whilst most physicians of the old school, imitating in a general manner the efforts of crude, unaided nature for its own relief, carried out in their practice these derivations of merely hypothetical utility, just as they judged expedient (guided by some imaginary indication), others, aiming at a higher object, undertook designedly to promote the efforts of the vital force to aid itself by evacuations and antagonistic metatases, as seen in diseases, and by way of lending it a helping hand, to increase still more these derivations and evacuations; and they believed that by this hurtful procedure they were acting duce natura, and might justly claim the title of minister naturae.

As the evacuations effected by the natural powers of the patient in chronic diseases are not infrequently the precursors of alleviations – though only of a temporary character – of troublesome symptoms, violent pains, paralyses, spasms, etc., so the old school imagined these derivations to be the true way of curing diseases, and endeavored to promote, maintain and even increase such evacuations. But they did not perceive that all these evacuations and excretions (pseudo-crises) produced by nature when left to herself were, in chronic diseases, only palliative, transient alleviations which, far from contributing to a real cure, on the contrary, rather aggravate the original, internal dyscrasia, by the waste of strength and juices they occasioned. No one ever saw a chronic patient recover his health permanently by such efforts of crude nature, nor any chronic disease cured by such evacuations effected by the organism. On the contrary, in such cases the original dyscrasia is always perceptibly aggravated, after alleviations, whose duration always becomes shorter and shorter; the bad attacks recur more frequently and more severely in spite of the continuation of the evacuations. In like manner, on the occurrence of symptoms excited by an internal chronic affection that threaten to destroy life, when nature left to its own resources, cannot help herself in any other way than by the production of external local symptoms, in order to avert the danger from parts indispensable to life and direct it to tissues of less vital importance (metastasis), these operations of the energetic but unintelligent, unreasoning and improvident vital force conduce to anything but genuine relief or recovery; they only silence in a palliative manner, for a short time, the dangerous internal affection at the cost of a large portion of the humours and of the strength, without diminishing the original disease by a hair's breadth; they can, at the most, only retard the fatal termination which is inevitable without true homoeopathic treatment.

22. Equally inefficacious are those produced artificially.

The allopathy of the old school not only greatly overrated these efforts of the crude automatic power of nature, but completely misjudged them, falsely considered them to be truly curative, and endeavored to increase and promote them, vainly imagining that thereby they might perhaps succeed in annihilating and radically curing the whole disease. When, in chronic diseases, the vital force seemed to silence this or that troublesome symptom of the internal affection by the production, for example, of some humid cutaneous eruption, then the servant of the crude power of nature (minister naturae) applied to the discharging surface a cantharides plaster or an exutory (mezereum), in order, *duce natura*, to draw still more moisture from the skin, and thus to promote and to assist natures object – the cure (by the removal of the morbific matter from the body?); but when the effect of the remedy was too violent, the eczema already of long standing, and the system too irritable, he increased the external affection to a great degree without the slightest advantage, to the original disease, and aggravated the pains, which deprived the patient of sleep and depressed his strength (and sometimes even developed a malignant febrile erysipelas); or if the effect upon the local affection (still recent, perhaps) was of milder character, he thereby repelled from its seat, by a species of ill-applied external homoeopathy, the local symptom which had been established by nature on the skin for the relief of the internal disease, thus renewing the more dangerous internal malady, and by this repulsion of the local symptom compelling the vital force to effect a transference of a worse form of morbid action to other and more important parts, the patient became affected with dangerous ophthalmia, or deafness, or spasms of the stomach, or epileptic convulsions, or attacks of asthma or apoplexy, or mental derangement, etc., in place of the repelled local disease.

23. Natural effects of the repulsion of these local symptoms – effects that are often regarded by the allopathic physician as fresh diseases of quite a different kind.

When the diseased natural force propelled blood into the veins of the rectum or anus (blind h¾morrhoids), the minister natura, under the same delusive idea of assisting the vital force in its curative efforts, applied leeches, often in large numbers, in order to give an outlet to the blood there – with but brief, often scarcely noteworthy, relief, but thereby weakening the body and occasioning still greater congestions in those parts, without the slightest diminution of the original disease.

In almost all cases in which the diseased vital force endeavored to subdue the violence of a dangerous internal malady by evacuating blood by means of vomiting, coughing, etc., the old school physician, *duce natura,* made haste to assist these supposed salutary efforts of nature, and performed a copious venesection, which was invariably productive of injurious consequences and palpable weakening of the body. In cases of frequently occurring chronic nausea, he produced, with the view of furthering the intentions of nature, copious evacuations of the stomach, by means of powerful emetics – never with a good result, often with bad, not infrequently dangerous and even fatal consequences.

The vital force, in order to relieve the internal malady, sometimes produces indolent enlargements of the external glands, and he thinks to forward the intentions of nature, in his assumed character of her servant, when, by the use of all sorts of heating embrocations and plasters, he causes them to inflame, so that, when the abscess is ripe, he may incise it and let out the bad morbific matter (?)

Experience has shown, hundreds of times, that lasting evil almost invariably results from such a plan.

And having often noticed slight amelioration of the severe symptoms of chronic diseases to result from spontaneous night sweats or frequent liquid stools, he imagines himself bound to obey these hints of nature (*duce natura*), and to promote them, by instituting and maintaining a complete course of sweating treatment or by the employment of so-called gentle laxatives for years, in order to promote and increase these efforts of nature (of the vital force of the unintelligent organism), which he thinks tend to the cure of the whole chronic affection, and thus to free the patient more speedily and certainly from his disease (the matter of his disease?).

But he thereby always produces quite the contrary result: aggravation of the original disease.

In conformity with this preconceived by unfounded idea, the old school physician goes on thus promoting the efforts of the diseased and increasing those derivations and evacuations in the patient which never lead to the desired end, but are always disastrous, without being aware that all the local affections, evacuations, and seemingly derivative efforts, set up and continued by the unintelligent vital force when left to its own resources, for the relief of the original chronic disease, are actually the disease itself, the phenomena of the whole disease, for the totality of which, properly speaking, the only efficacious remedy, and the one, moreover, that will act in the most direct manner, is a homoeopathic medicine, chosen on account of its similarity of action.

Note

24. In direct opposition to this treatment, the old school not infrequently indulged themselves in the very reverse of this: thus when the efforts of the vital force for the relief of the internal disease by evacuations and the production of local symptoms on the exterior of the body became troublesome, they capriciously suppressed them by their repercutients and repellents, they subdued chronic pains, sleeplessness and diarrhoea of long standing by doses of opium pushed to a dangerous extent; vomitings by effervescent saline draughts; foetid perspiration of the feet by cold footbaths and astringent applications; eruptions on the skin by preparations of lead and zinc; they checked uterine haemorrhage by injections of vinegar; colliquative perspiration by alum; nocturnal seminal emissions by the free use of camphor; frequent attacks of flushes of heat in the body and face by nitre vegetable acids and sulphuric acid; bleeding of the nose by plugging the nostrils with dossils of lint soaked in alcohol or astringent fluids; they dried up discharging ulcers on the legs, established by the vital power for the relief of great internal suffering with the oxides of lead and zinc, etc.

The Aphorisms

§ 1

The physician's high and only mission is to restore the sick to health, to cure, as it is termed.1

1 His mission is not, however, to construct so-called systems, by interweaving empty speculations and hypotheses concerning the internal essential nature of the vital processes and the mode in which diseases originate in the interior of the organism, (whereon so many physicians have hitherto ambitiously wasted their talents and their time); nor is it to attempt to give countless explanations regarding the phenomena in diseases and their proximate cause (which must ever remain concealed), wrapped in unintelligible words and an inflated abstract mode of expression, which should sound very learned in order to astonish the ignorant – whilst sick humanity sighs in vain for aid. Of such learned reveries (to which the name of theoretic medicine is given, and for which special professorships are instituted) we have had quite enough, and it is now high time that all who call themselves physicians should at length cease to deceive suffering mankind with mere talk, and begin now, instead, for once to act, that is, really to help and to cure.

§ 2

The highest ideal of cure is rapid, gentle and permanent restoration of the health, or removal and annihilation of the disease in its whole extent, in the shortest, most reliable, and most harmless way, on easily comprehensible principles.

§ 3

If the physician clearly perceives what is to be cured in diseases, that is to say, in every individual case of disease (knowledge of disease, indication), if he clearly perceives what is curative in medicines, that is to say, in each individual medicine (knowledge of medical powers), and if he knows how to adapt, according to clearly defined principles, what is curative in medicines to what he has discovered to be undoubtedly morbid in the patient, so that the recovery must ensue – to adapt it, as well in respect to the suitability of the medicine most appropriate according to its mode of action to the case before him (choice of the remedy, the medicine indicated), as also in respect to the exact mode of preparation and quantity of it required (proper dose), and the proper period for repeating the dose; – if, finally, he knows the obstacles to recovery in each case and is aware how to remove them, so that the restoration may be permanent, then he understands how to treat judiciously and rationally, and he is a true practitioner of the healing art.

§ 4

He is likewise a preserver of health if he knows the things that derange health and cause disease, and how to remove them from persons in health.

§ 5

Useful to the physician in assisting him to cure are the particulars of the most probable exciting cause of the acute disease, as also the most significant points in the whole history of the chronic disease, to enable him to discover its fundamental cause, which is generally due to a chronic miasm. In these investigations, the ascertainable physical constitution of the patient (especially when the disease is chronic), his moral and intellectual character, his occupation, mode of living and habits, his social and domestic relations, his age, sexual function, etc., are to be taken into consideration.

§ 6 Fifth Edition

The unprejudiced observer – well aware of the futility of transcendental speculations which can receive no confirmation from experience – be his powers of penetration ever so great, takes note of nothing in every individual disease, except the changes in the health of the body and of the mind (morbid phenomena, accidents, symptoms) which can be perceived externally by means of the senses; that is to say, he notices only the deviations from the former healthy state of the now diseased individual, which are felt by the patient himself, remarked by those around him and observed by the physician. All these perceptible signs represent the disease in its whole extent, that is, together they form the true and only conceivable portrait of the disease. [1]

§ 6 Sixth Edition

The unprejudiced observer – well aware of the futility of transcendental speculations which can receive no confirmation from experience – be his powers of penetration ever so great, takes note of nothing in every individual disease, except the changes in the health of the body and of the mind (morbid phenomena, accidents, symptoms) which can be perceived externally by means of the senses; that is to say, he notices only the deviations from the former healthy state of the now diseased individual, which are felt by the patient himself, remarked by those around him and observed by the physician. All these perceptible signs represent the disease in its whole extent, that is, together they form the true and only conceivable portrait of the disease. [1]

Is not, then, that which is cognizable by the senses in diseases through the phenomena it displays, the disease itself in the eyes of the physician, since he never can see the spiritual being that produces the disease, the vital force? nor is it necessary that he should see it, but only that he should ascertain its morbid actions, in order that he may thereby be enabled to cure the disease. What else will the old school search for in the hidden interior of the organism, as a prima causa morbi, whilst they reject as an object of cure and contemptuously despise the sensible and manifest representation of the disease, the symptoms, that so plainly address themselves to us? What else do they wish to cure in disease but these?

§ 7

Now, as in a disease, from which no manifest exciting or maintaining cause (causa occasionalis) has to be removed [2], we can perceive nothing but the morbid symptoms, it must (regard being had to the possibility of a miasm, and attention paid to the accessory circumstances, § 5) be the symptoms alone by which the disease demands and points to the remedy suited to relieve it – and, moreover, the totality of these its symptoms, of this outwardly reflected picture of the internal essence of the disease, that is, of the affection of the vital force, must be the principal, or the sole means, whereby the disease can make known what remedy it requires – the only thing that can determine the choice of the most appropriate remedy – and thus, in a word, the totality [3] of the symptoms must be the principal, indeed the only thing the physician has to take note of in every case of disease and to remove by means of his art, in order that it shall be cured and transformed into health.

§ 8
It is not conceivable, not can it be proved by any experience in the world, that, after removal of all the symptoms of the disease and of the entire collection of the perceptible phenomena, there should or could remain anything else besides health, or that the morbid alteration in the interior could remain uneradicated. [4]

§ 9
In the healthy condition of man, the spiritual vital force (autocracy), the dynamis that animates the material body (organism), rules with unbounded sway, and retains all the parts of the organism in admirable, harmonious, vital operation, as regards both sensations and functions, so that our indwelling, reason-gifted mind can freely employ this living, healthy instrument for the higher purpose of our existence.

§ 10 Fifth Edition
The material organism, without the vital force, is capable of no sensation, no function, no self-preservation [5], it derives all sensation and performs all the functions of life solely by means of the immaterial being (the vital force) which animates the material organism in health and in disease.

§ 10 Sixth Edition
The material organism, without the vital force, is capable of no sensation, no function, no self-preservation [5], it derives all sensation and performs all the functions of life solely by means of the immaterial being (the vital principle) which animates the material organism in health and in disease.

§ 11 Fifth Edition
When a person falls ill, it is only this spiritual, self acting (automatic) vital force, everywhere present in his organism, that is primarily deranged by the dynamic [6] influence upon it of a morbific agent inimical to life; it is only the vital force, deranged to such an abnormal state, that can furnish the organism with its disagreeable sensations, and incline it to the irregular processes which we call disease; for, as a power invisible in itself, and only cognizable by its effects on the organism, its morbid derangement only makes itself known by the manifestation of disease in the sensations and functions of those parts of the organism exposed to the senses of the observer and physician, that is, by morbid symptoms, and in no other way can it make itself known.

§ 11 Sixth Edition
When a person falls ill, it is only this spiritual, self acting (automatic) vital force, everywhere present in his organism, that is primarily deranged by the dynamic [6] influence upon it of a morbific agent inimical to life; it is only the vital force, deranged to such an abnormal state, that can furnish the organism with its disagreeable sensations, and incline it to the irregular processes which we call disease; for, as a power invisible in itself, and only cognizable by its effects on the organism, its morbid derangement only makes itself known by the manifestation

of disease in the sensations and functions of those parts of the organism exposed to the senses of the observer and physician, that is, by morbid symptoms, and in no other way can it make itself known. [7]

§ 12 Fifth Edition

It is the morbidly affected vital force alone that produces disease [8], so that the morbid phenomena perceptible to our senses express at the same time all the internal change, that is to say, the whole morbid derangement of the internal dynamis; in a word, they reveal the whole disease; consequently, also, the disappearance under treatment of all the morbid phenomena and of all the morbid alterations that differ from the healthy vital operations, certainly affects and necessarily implies the restoration of the integrity of the vital force and, therefore, the recovered health of the whole organism.

§ 12 Sixth Edition

It is the morbidly affected vital energy alone that produces disease [8], so that the morbid phenomena perceptible to our senses express at the same time all the internal change, that is to say, the whole morbid derangement of the internal dynamis; in a word, they reveal the whole disease; consequently, also, the disappearance under treatment of all the morbid phenomena and of all the morbid alterations that differ from the healthy vital operations, certainly affects and necessarily implies the restoration of the integrity of the vital force and, therefore, the recovered health of the whole organism.

§ 13

Therefore disease (that does not come within the province of manual surgery) considered, as it is by the allopathists, as a thing separate from the living whole, from the organism and its animating vital force, and hidden in the interior, be it ever so subtle a character, is an absurdity, that could only be imagined by minds of a materialistic stamp, and has for thousands of years given to the prevailing system of medicine all those pernicious impulses that have made it a truly mischievous (non-healing) art.

§ 14

There is, in the interior of man, nothing morbid that is curable and no invisible morbid alteration that is curable which does not make itself known to the accurately observing physicians by means of morbid signs and symptoms – an arrangement in perfect conformity with the infinite goodness of the all-wise Preserver of human life.

§ 15 Fifth Edition

The affection of the morbidly deranged, spirit-like dynamis (vital force) that animates our body in the invisible interior, and the totality of the outwardly cognizable symptoms produced by it in the organism and representing the existing malady, constitute a whole; they are one and the same. The organism is indeed the material instrument of the life, but it is not conceivable without the animation imparted to it by the instinctively perceiving and regulating vital force (just as the vital force is not conceivable without the organism), consequently the two together constitute a unity, although in thought our mind separates this unity into two distinct conceptions for the sake of facilitating the comprehension of it.

§ 15 Sixth Edition

The affection of the morbidly deranged, spirit-like dynamis (vital force) that animates our body in the invisible interior, and the totality of the outwardly cognizable symptoms produced by it in the organism and representing the existing malady, constitute a whole; they are one and the same. The organism is indeed the material instrument of the life, but it is not conceivable without the animation imparted to it by the instinctively perceiving and regulating dynamis, just as the vital force is not conceivable without the organism, consequently the two together constitute a unity, although in thought our mind separates this unity into two distinct conceptions for the sake of easy comprehension.

§ 16 Fifth Edition

Our vital force, as a spirit-like dynamis, cannot be attacked and affected by injurious influences on the healthy organism caused by the external inimical forces that disturb the harmonious play of life, otherwise than in a spirit-like (dynamic) way, and in like manner, all such morbid derangements (diseases) cannot be removed from it by the physician in any other way than by the spirit-like (dynamic [9], virtual) alterative powers of the serviceable medicines acting upon our spirit-like vital force, which perceives them through the medium of the sentient faculty of the nerves everywhere present in the organism, so that it is only by their dynamic action on the vital force that remedies are able to re-establish and do actually re-establish health and vital harmony, after the changes in the health of the patient cognizable by our senses (the totality of the symptoms) have revealed the disease to the carefully observing and investigating physician as fully as was requisite in order to enable him to cure it.

§ 16 Sixth Edition

Our vital force, as a spirit-like dynamis, cannot be attacked and affected by injurious influences on the healthy organism caused by the external inimical forces that disturb the harmonious play of life, otherwise than in a spirit-like (dynamic) way, and in like manner, all such morbid derangements (diseases) cannot be removed from it by the physician in any other way than by the spirit-like (dynamic [9], virtual) alterative powers of the serviceable medicines acting upon our spirit-like vital force, which perceives them through the medium of the sentient faculty of the nerves everywhere present in the organism, so that it is only by their dynamic action on the vital force that remedies are able to re-establish and do actually re-establish health and vital harmony, after the changes in the health of the patient cognizable by our senses (the totality of the symptoms) have revealed the disease to the carefully observing and investigating physician as fully as was requisite in order to enable him to cure it.

§ 17 Fifth Edition

Now, as in the cure effected by the removal of the whole of the perceptible signs and symptoms of the disease the internal alteration of the vital force to which the disease is due – consequently the whole of the disease – is at the same time removed, [10] it follows that the physician has only to remove the whole of the symptoms in order, at the same time, to abrogate and annihilate the internal change, that is to say, the morbid derangement of the vital force – consequently the totality of the disease, the disease itself. [11] But when the disease is annihilated the health is restored, and this is the highest, the sole aim of the physician who knows the true object of his mission, which consists not in learned – sounding prating, but in giving aid to the sick.

§ 17 Sixth Edition
Now, as in the cure effected by the removal of the whole of the perceptible signs and symptoms of the disease the internal alteration of the vital principle to which the disease is due – consequently the whole of the disease – is at the same time removed, [10] it follows that the physician has only to remove the whole of the symptoms in order, at the same time, to abrogate and annihilate the internal change, that is to say, the morbid derangement of the vital force – consequently the totality of the disease, the disease itself. [11] But when the disease is annihilated the health is restored, and this is the highest, the sole aim of the physician who knows the true object of his mission, which consists not in learned – sounding prating, but in giving aid to the sick.

§ 18 Fifth Edition
From this indubitable truth, that besides the totality of the symptoms nothing can by any means be discovered in disease wherewith they could express their need of aid, it follows undeniably that the sum of all the symptoms in each individual case of disease must be the sole indication, the sole guide to direct us in the choice of a remedy.

§ 18 Sixth Edition
From this indubitable truth, that besides the totality of the symptoms with consideration of the accompanying modalities (§ 5) nothing can by any means be discovered in disease wherewith they could express their need of aid, it follows undeniably that the sum of all the symptoms and conditions in each individual case of disease must be the sole indication, the sole guide to direct us in the choice of a remedy.

§ 19
Now, as diseases are nothing more than alterations in the state of health of the healthy individual which express themselves by morbid signs, and the cure is also only possible by a change to the healthy condition of the state of health of the diseased individual, it is very evident that medicines could never cure disease if they did not possess the power of altering man's state of health which depends on sensations and functions; indeed, that their curative power must be owing solely to this power they possess of altering man's state of health.

§ 20 Fifth edition
This spirit-like power to alter man's state of health (and hence to cure diseases) which lies hidden in the inner nature of medicines can never be discovered by us by a mere effort of reason; it is only by experience of the phenomena it displays when acting on the state of health of man that we can become clearly cognizant of it.

§ 20 Sixth edition
This spirit-like power to alter man's state of health (and hence to cure diseases) which lies hidden in the inner nature of medicines can in itself never be discovered by us by a mere effort of reason; it is only by experience of the phenomena it displays when acting on the state of health of man that we can become clearly cognizant of it.

§ 21

Now, as it is undeniable that the curative principle in medicines is not in itself perceptible, and as in pure experiments with medicines conducted by the most accurate observers, nothing can be observed that can constitute them medicines or remedies except that power of causing distinct alterations in the state of health of the human body, and particularly in that of the healthy individual, and of exciting in him various definite morbid symptoms; so it follows that when medicines act as remedies, they can only bring their curative property into play by means of this their power of altering man's state of health by the production of peculiar symptoms; and that, therefore, we have only to rely on the morbid phenomena which the medicines produce in the healthy body as the sole possible revelation of their in-dwelling curative power, in order to learn what disease-producing power, and at the same time what disease-curing power, each individual medicine possesses.

§ 22 Fifth Edition

But as nothing is to be observed in diseases that must be removed in order to change them into health besides the totality of their signs and symptoms, and likewise medicines can show nothing curative besides their tendency to produce morbid symptoms in healthy persons and to remove them in diseased persons; it follows, on the one hand, that medicines only become remedies and capable of annihilating disease, because the medicinal substance, by exciting certain effects and symptoms, that is to say, by producing a certain artificial morbid state, removes and abrogates the symptoms already present, to wit, the natural morbid state we wish to cure. On the other hand, it follows that, for the totality of the symptoms of the disease to be cured, a medicine must be sought which (according as experience shall prove whether the morbid symptoms are most readily, certainly, and permanently removed and changed into health by similar or opposite medicinal symptoms [12]) has a tendency to produce similar or opposite symptoms.

§ 22 Sixth Edition

But as nothing is to be observed in diseases that must be removed in order to change them into health besides the totality of their signs and symptoms, and likewise medicines can show nothing curative besides their tendency to produce morbid symptoms in healthy persons and to remove them in diseased persons; it follows, on the one hand, that medicines only become remedies and capable of annihilating disease, because the medicinal substance, by exciting certain effects and symptoms, that is to say, by producing a certain artificial morbid state, removes and abrogates the symptoms already present, to wit, the natural morbid state we wish to cure. On the other hand, it follows that, for the totality of the symptoms of the disease to be cured, a medicine must be sought which (according as experience shall prove whether the morbid symptoms are most readily, certainly, and permanently removed and changed into health by similar or opposite medicinal symptoms [13]) have the greatest tendency to produce similar or opposite symptoms.

§ 23

All pure experience, however, and all accurate research convince us that persistent symptoms of disease are far from being removed and annihilated by opposite symptoms of medicines (as in the antipathic, enantiopathic or palliative method), that, on the contrary, after transient, apparent alleviation, they break forth again, only with increased intensity, and become manifestly aggravated (see § 58 – 62 and 69).

§ 24
There remains, therefore, no other mode of employing medicines in diseases that promises to be of service besides the homoeopathic, by means of which we seek, for the totality of the symptoms of the case of disease, a medicine which among all medicines (whose pathogenetic effects are known from having been tested in healthy individuals) has the power and the tendency to produce an artificial morbid state most similar to that of the case of disease in question.

§ 25
Now, however, in all careful trials, pure experience, [14] the sole and infallible oracle of the healing art, teaches us that actually that medicine which, in its action on the healthy human body, has demonstrated its power of producing the greatest number of symptoms similar to those observable in the case of disease under treatment, does also, in doses of suitable potency and attenuation, rapidly, radically and permanently remove the totality of the symptoms of this morbid state, that is to say (§ 6 – 16), the whole disease present, and change it into health; and that all medicines cure, without exception, those diseases whose symptoms most nearly resemble their own, and leave none of them uncured.

§ 26
This depends on the following homoeopathic law of nature which was sometimes, indeed, vaguely surmised but not hitherto fully recognized, and to which is due every real cure that has ever taken place:

A weaker dynamic affection is permanently extinguished in the living organism by a stronger one, if the latter (whilst differing in kind) is very similar to the former in its manifestations. [15]

§ 27
The curative power of medicines, therefore, depends on their symptoms, similar to the disease but superior to it in strength (§ 12 – 26), so that each individual case of disease is most surely, radically, rapidly and permanently annihilated and removed only by a medicine capable of producing (in the human system) in the most similar and complete manner the totality of its symptoms, which at the same time are stronger than the disease.

§ 28
As this natural law of cure manifests itself in every pure experiment and every true observation in the world, the fact is consequently established; it matters little what may be scientific explanation of how it takes place; and I do not attach much importance to the attempts made to explain it. But the following view seems to commend itself as the most probable one, as it is founded on premises derived from experience.

§ 29 Fifth Edition
As every disease (not strictly belonging to the domain of surgery) depends only on a peculiar morbid derangement of our vital force in sensations and functions, when a homoeopathic cure of the vital force deranged by natural disease is accomplished by the administration of a medicinal agent selected on account of an accurate similarity of symptoms, a somewhat stronger, similar, artificial mor-

bid affection is brought into contact with and, as it were, pushed into the place of the weaker, similar, natural morbid irritation, against which the instinctive vital force, now merely (though in a stronger degree) medicinally diseased, is then compelled to direct an increased amount of energy, but, on account of the shorter duration of the action [16] of the medicinal agent that now morbidly affects it, the vital force soon overcomes this, and as it was in the first instance relieved from the natural morbid affection, so it is now at last freed from the substituted artificial (medicinal) one, and hence is enable again to carry on healthily the vital operations of the organism. This highly probable explanation of the process rests on the following axioms.

§ 29 Sixth Edition

As every disease (not entirely surgical) consists only in a special, morbid, dynamic alteration of our vital energy (of the principle of life) manifested in sensation and motion, so in every homoeopathic cure this principle of life dynamically altered by natural disease is seized through the administration of medicinal potency selected exactly according to symptom-similarity by a somewhat stronger, similar artificial disease-manifestation. By this the feeling of the natural (weaker) dynamic disease-manifestation ceases and disappears. This disease-manifestation no longer exists for the principle of life which is now occupied and governed merely by the stronger, artificial disease-manifestation. This artificial disease-manifestation has soon spent its force and leaves the patient free from disease, cured. The dynamis, thus freed, can now continue to carry life on in health. This most highly probable process rests upon the following propositions.

§ 30 Fifth Edition

The human body appears to admit of being much more powerfully affected in its health by medicines (partly because we have the regulation of the dose in our own power) than by natural morbid stimuli – for natural diseases are cured and overcome by suitable medicines.

§ 30 Sixth Edition

The human body appears to admit of being much more powerfully affected in its health by medicines (partly because we have the regulation of the dose in our own power) than by natural morbid stimuli – for natural diseases are cured and overcome by suitable medicines. [17]

§ 31

The inimical forces, partly psychical, partly physical, to which our terrestrial existence is exposed, which are termed morbific noxious agents, do not possess the power of morbidly deranging the health of man unconditionally; [18] but we are made ill by them only when our organism is sufficiently disposed and susceptible to attack of the morbific cause that may be present, and to be altered in its health, deranged and made to undergo abnormal sensations and functions – hence they do not produce disease in every one nor at all times.

§ 32

But it is quite otherwise with the artificial morbific agents which we term medicines. Every real medicine, namely, acts at all times, under all circumstances, on every living human being, and produces in him its peculiar symptoms (distinctly perceptible, if the dose be large enough), so that evidently every living human organism is liable to be affected, and, as it were, inoculated with the medicinal disease at all times, and absolutely (unconditionally), which, as before said, is by no means the case with the natural diseases.

§ 33
In accordance with this fact, it is undeniably shown by all experience [19] that the living organism is much more disposed and has a greater liability to be acted on, and to have its health deranged by medicinal powers, than by morbific noxious agents and infectious miasms, or, in order words, that the morbific noxious agents possess a power of morbidly deranging man's health that is subordinate and conditional, often very conditional; whilst medicinal agents have an absolute unconditional power, greatly superior to the former.

§ 34 Fifth Edition
The greater strength of the artificial diseases producible by medicines is, however, not the sole cause of their power to cure natural disease. In order that they may effect a cure, it is before all things requisite that they should be capable of producing in the human body an artificial disease as similar as possible to the disease to be cured, in order, by means of this similarity, conjoined with its somewhat greater strength, to substitute themselves for the natural morbid affection, and thereby deprive the latter of all influence upon the vital force. This is so true, that no previously existing disease can be cured, even by Nature herself, by the accession of a new dissimilar disease, be it ever so strong, and just as little can it be cured by medical treatment with drugs which are incapable of producing a similar morbid condition in the healthy body.

§ 34 Sixth Edition
The greater strength of the artificial diseases producible by medicines is, however, not the sole cause of their power to cure natural disease. In order that they may effect a cure, it is before all things requisite that they should be capable of producing in the human body an artificial disease as similar as possible to the disease to be cured, which, with somewhat increased power, transforms to a very similar morbid state the instinctive life principle, which in itself is incapable of any reflection or act of memory. It not only obscures, but extinguishes and thereby annihilates the derangement caused by the natural disease. This is so true, that no previously existing disease can be cured, even by Nature herself, by the accession of a new dissimilar disease, be it ever so strong, and just as little can it be cured by medical treatment with drugs which are incapable of producing a similar morbid condition in the healthy body.

§ 35
In order to illustrate this, we shall consider in three different cases, as well what happens in nature when two dissimilar natural diseases meet to in one person, as also the result of the ordinary medical treatment of diseases with unsuitable allopathic drugs, which are incapable of producing an artificial morbid condition similar to the disease to be cured, whereby it will appear that even Nature herself is unable to remove a dissimilar disease already present by one that is unhomoeopathic, even though it be stronger, and just as little is the unhomoeopathic employment of even the strongest medicines ever capable of curing any disease whatsoever.

§ 36

I. If the two dissimilar diseases meeting together in the human being be of equal strength, or still more if the older one be the stronger, the new disease will be repelled by the old one from the body and not allowed to affect it. A patient suffering from a severe chronic disease will not be infected by a moderate autumnal dysentery or other epidemic disease. The plague of the Levant, according to Larry, [20] does not break out where scurvy is prevalent, and persons suffering from eczema are not infected by it. Rachitis, Jenner alleges, prevents vaccination from taking effect. Those suffering from pulmonary consumption are not liable to be attacked by epidemic fevers of a not very violent character, according to Von Hildenbrand.

§ 37 Fifth Edition

So, also under ordinary medical treatment, an old chronic disease remains uncured and unaltered if it is treated according to the common allopathic method, that is to say, with medicines that are incapable of producing in healthy individuals a state of health similar to the disease, even though the treatment should last for years and is not of too violent character. This is daily witnessed in practice, it is therefore unnecessary to give any illustrative examples.

§ 37 Sixth Edition

So, also under ordinary medical treatment, an old chronic disease remains uncured and unaltered if it is treated according to the common allopathic method, that is to say, with medicines that are incapable of producing in healthy individuals a state of health similar to the disease, even though the treatment should last for years and is not of too violent character. [21] This is daily witnessed in practice, it is therefore unnecessary to give any illustrative examples.

§ 38

II. Or the new dissimilar disease is the stronger. In this case the disease under which the patient originally labored, being the weaker, will be kept back and suspended by the accession of the stronger one, until the latter shall have run its course or been cured, and then the old one reappears uncured. Two children affected with a kind of epilepsy remained free from epileptic attacks after infection with ringworm (tinea) but as soon as the eruption on the head was gone the epilepsy returned just as before, as Tulpius [22] observed. The itch, as Schopf [23] saw, disappeared on the occurrence of the scurvy, but after the cure of the latter it again broke out. So, also the pulmonary phthisis remained stationary when the patient was attacked by a violent typhus, but went on again after the latter had run its course. [24] If mania occur in a consumptive patient, the phthisis with all its symptoms is removed by the former; but if that go off, the phthisis returns immediately and proves fatal. [25] When measles and smallpox are prevalent at the same time, and both attack the same child, the measles that had already broken out is generally checked by the smallpox that came somewhat later; nor does the measles resume its course until after the cure of the smallpox; but it not infrequently happens that the inoculated smallpox is suspended for four days by the supervention of the measles, as observed by Manget, [26] after the desquamation of which the smallpox completes its course. Even when the inoculation of the smallpox had taken effect for six days, and the measles then broke out, the inflammation of the inoculation remained stationary and the smallpox did not ensue until the measles had completed its regular course of seven days. [27] In an epidemic of measles, that disease attacked many individuals on the fourth or fifth day after the inoculation of smallpox and prevented the development of the smallpox until it had completed its own course, whereupon the smallpox appeared and proceeded regularly to its termination. [28] The true, smooth, erysipelatous-looking scarlatina of Sydenham, with sore throat, was checked on the fourth day by the eruption of cow-pox, which ran its regular course, and not till it was ended did the scarlatina again establish itself; but on another occasion, as both diseases seem to be of equal strength, the cow-pox was suspended on the eighth day by the supervention of the true, smooth scarlatina of Sydenham, [29] and the red areola of the former disappeared until the scarlatina was gone, wherein the cow-pox immediately resumed its course, and went on its regular termination. [30] The measles suspended the cow-pox; on the eighth day, when the cow-pox had nearly attained its climax, the measles broke out; the cow-pox now remained stationary, and did not resume and complete its course until the desquamation of the measles, had taken place, so that on the sixteenth day it presented the appearance it otherwise would have shown on the tenth day, as Kortum [31] observed.

Even after the measles had broken out the cow-pox inoculation took effect, but did not run its course until these measles had disappeared, as Kortum likewise witnessed. [32]

I myself saw the mumps (angina parotidea) immediately disappear when the cow-pox inoculation had taken effect and had nearly attained its height; it was not until the complete termination of the cow-pox and the disappearance of its red areola that this febrile tumefaction of the parotid and submaxillary glands, that is caused by a peculiar miasm, reappeared and ran its regular course of seven days.

And thus it is with all dissimilar disease; the stronger suspends the weaker (when they do not complicate one another, which is seldom the case with acute disease), but they never cure one another.

§ 39

Now the adherents of the ordinary school of medicine saw all this for so many centuries; they saw that Nature herself cannot cure any disease by the accession of another, be it ever so strong, if the new disease be dissimilar to that already present in the body. What shall we think of them, that they nevertheless went on treating chronic disease with allopathic remedies, namely, with medicines and prescriptions capable of producing God knows what morbid state – almost invariably, however, one dissimilar to the disease to be cured? And even though physicians did not hitherto observe nature attentively, the miserable results of their treatment should have taught them that they were pursuing an inappropriate, a false path. Did they not perceive when they employed, as was their custom, and aggressive allopathic treatment in a chronic disease, that thereby they only created an artificial disease dissimilar to the original one, which, as long as it was kept up, merely held in abeyance, merely suppressed, merely suspended the original disease, which latter, however, always returned, and must return, as soon as the diminished strength of the patient no longer admitted of a continuance of the allopathic attacks on the life? Thus the itch exanthema certainly disappears very soon from the skin under the employment of violent purgatives, frequently repeated; but when the patient can no longer stand the factitious (dissimilar) disease of the bowels, and can take no more purgatives, then either the cutaneous eruption breaks out as before, or the internal psora displays itself in some bad symptom, and the patient, in addition to his undiminished original disease, has to endure the misery of a painful ruined digestion and impaired strength to boot. So, also, when the ordinary physicians keep up artificial ulcerations of the skin and issues on the exterior of the body, with the view of thereby eradicating a chronic disease, they can NEVER cure them by that means, as such artificial cutaneous ulcers are quite alien and allopathic to the internal affection; but inasmuch as the irritation produced by several tissues is at least sometimes a stronger (dissimilar) disease than the indwelling malady, the latter is thereby sometimes silenced and suspended for a week or two. But it is only suspended, and that for a very short time, while the patient's powers are gradually worn out. Epilepsy, suppressed for many years by means of issues, invariably recurred, and in an aggravated form, when they were allowed to heal up, as Pechlin [33] and others testify. But purgatives for itch, and issues for epilepsy, cannot be more heterogeneous, more dissimilar deranging agents – cannot be more allopathic, more exhausting modes of treatment – than are the customary prescriptions, composed of unknown ingredients, used in ordinary practice for the other nameless, innumerable forms of disease. These likewise do nothing but debilitate, and only suppress or suspend the malady for a short time without being able to cure it, and when used for a long time always add a new morbid state to the old disease.

§ 40

III. Or the new disease, after having long acted on the organism, at length joins the old one that is dissimilar to it, and forms with it a complex disease, so that each of them occupies a particular locality in the organism, namely, the organs peculiarly adapted for it, and, as it were, only the place specially belonging to it, while it leaves the rest to the other disease that is dissimilar to it. Thus a syphilitic patient may become psoric, and vice versa. As two disease dissimilar to each other, they cannot remove, cannot cure one another. At first the venereal symptoms are kept in abeyance and suspended when the psoric eruption begins to appear; in course of time, however (as the syphilis is at least as strong as the psora), the two join together, [34] that is, each involves those parts of the organism only which are most adapted for it, and the patient is thereby rendered more diseased and more difficult to cure.

When two dissimilar acute infectious diseases meet, as, for example, smallpox and measles, the one usually suspends the other, as has been before observed; yet there have also been severe epidemics of this kind, where, in rare cases, two dissimilar acute diseases occurred simultaneously in one and the same body, and for a short time combined, as it were, with each other. During an epidemic, in which smallpox and measles were prevalent at the same time, among three hundred cases (in which these diseases avoided or suspended one another, and measles attacked patients twenty days after the smallpox broke out, the smallpox, however, from seventeen to eighteen days after the appearance of the measles, so that the first disease had previously completed its regular course) there was yet one single case in which P. Russell [35] met with both these dissimilar diseases in one person at the same time. Rainey [36] witnessed the simultaneous occurrence of smallpox and measles in two girls. J. Maurice [37], in his whole practice, only observed two such cases. Similar cases are to be found in Ettmuller's [38] works, and in the writings of a few others.

Zencker [39] saw cow-pox run its regular course along with measles and along with purpura.

The cow-pox went on its course undisturbed during a mercurial treatment for syphilis, as Jenner saw.

§ 41 Fifth Edition

Much more frequent than the natural diseases associating with and complicating one another in the same body are the morbid complication resulting from the art of the ordinary practitioner, which the inappropriate medical treatment (the allopathic method) is apt to produce by the long-continued employment of unsuitable drugs. To the natural disease, which it is proposed to cure, there are then added, by the constant repetition of the unsuitable medical agent, the new, often very tedious, morbid conditions which might be anticipated from the peculiar powers of the drug; these gradually coalesce with and complicate the chronic malady which is dissimilar to them (which they were unable to cure by similarity of action, that is, homoeopathically), adding to the old disease a new, dissimilar, artificial malady of a chronic nature, and thus give the patient a double in place of a single disease, that is to say, render him much worse and more difficult to cure, often quite incurable. Many of the cases for which advice is asked in medical journals, as also the records of other cases in medical writings, attest the truth of this. Of a similar character are the frequent cases in which the venereal chancrous disease, complicated especially with psora or with the venereal chancrous disease, complicated especially with psora or with dyscrasia of condylomatous gonorrhoea, is not cured by long-continued or frequently repeated treatment with large doses of unsuitable mercurial preparations, but assumes its place in the organism beside the chronic mercurial affection1 that has been in the meantime gradually developed, and thus along with it often forms a hideous monster of complicated disease (under the general name of masked venereal disease), which then, when not quite incurable, can only be transformed into health with the greatest difficulty.

§ 41 Sixth Edition

Much more frequent than the natural diseases associating with and complicating one another in the same body are the morbid complication resulting from the art of the ordinary practitioner, which the inappropriate medical treatment (the allopathic method) is apt to produce by the long-continued employment of unsuitable drugs. To the natural disease, which it is proposed to cure, there are then added, by the constant repetition of the unsuitable medical agent, the new, often very tedious, morbid conditions corresponding to the nature of this agent; these gradually coalesce with and complicate the chronic malady which is dissimilar to them (which they were unable to cure by similarity of action, that is, homoeopathically), adding to the old disease a new, dissimilar, artificial malady of a chronic nature, and thus give the patient a double in place of a single disease, that is to say, render him much worse and more difficult to cure, often quite incurable. Many of the cases for which advice is asked in medical journals, as also the records of other cases in medical writings, attest the truth of this. Of a similar character are the frequent cases in which the venereal chancrous disease, complicated especially with psora or with the venereal chancrous disease, complicated especially with psora or with dyscrasia of condylomatous gonorrhoea, is not cured by long-continued or frequently repeated treatment with large doses of unsuitable mercurial preparations, but assumes its place in the organism beside the chronic mercurial affection [40] that has been in the meantime gradually developed, and thus along with it often forms a hideous monster of complicated disease (under the general name of masked venereal disease), which then, when not quite incurable, can only be transformed into health with the greatest difficulty.

§ 42

Nature herself permits, as has been stated, in some cases, the simultaneous occurrence of two (indeed, of three) natural disease in one and the same body. This complication, however, it must be remarked, happens only in the case of two dissimilar disease, which according to the eternal laws of nature do not remove, do not annihilate and cannot cure one another, but, as it seems, both (or all three) remain, as it were, separate in the organism, and each takes possession of the parts and systems peculiarly appropriate to it, which, on account of the want of resemblance of these maladies to each other, can very well happen without disparagement to the unity of life.

§ 43

Totally different, however, is the result when two similar disease meet together in the organism, that is to say, when to the disease already present a stronger similar one is added. In such cases we see how a cure can be effected by the operations of nature, and we get a lesson as to how man ought to cure.

§ 44 Fifth Edition

Two diseases similar to each other can neither (as is asserted of dissimilar disease in I) repel one another, nor (as has been shown of dissimilar disease in II) suspend on another, so that the old one shall return after the new one has run its course; and just as little can two similar disease (as has been demonstrated in III respecting dissimilar affections) exist beside each other in the same organism, or together form a double complex disease.

§ 44 Sixth Edition

Similar diseases can neither (as is asserted of dissimilar disease in I) repel one another, nor (as has been shown of dissimilar disease in II) suspend on another, so that the old one shall return after the new one has run its course; and just as little can two similar disease (as has been demonstrated in III respecting dissimilar affections) exist beside each other in the same organism, or together form a double complex disease.

§ 45 Fifth Edition

No! Two diseases, differing, it is true, in kind [41] but very similar in their phenomena and effects and in the sufferings and symptoms they severally produce, invariably annihilate one another whenever they meet together in the organism; the stronger disease namely, annihilates the weaker, and that for this simple reason, because the stronger morbific power when it invades the system, by reason of its similarity of action involves precisely the same part of the organism that were previously affected by the weaker morbid irritation, which, consequently, can no longer act on these parts, but is extinguished, [42] or (in other words) because, whenever the vital force, deranged by the primary disease, is more strongly attacked by the new, very similar, but stronger dynamic morbific power, it therefore now remains affected by the latter alone, whereby the original, similar but weaker disease must, as a mere dynamic power without material substratum, cease to exercise any further morbid influence on the vital force, consequently it must cease to exist.

§ 45 Sixth Edition

No! Two diseases, differing, it is true, in kind [41] but very similar in their phenomena and effects and in the sufferings and symptoms they severally produce, invariably annihilate one another whenever they meet together in the organism; the stronger disease namely, annihilates the weaker, and that for this simple reason, because the stronger morbific power when it invades the system, by reason of its similarity of action involves precisely the same part of the organism that were previously affected by the weaker morbid irritation, which, consequently, can no longer act on these parts, but is extinguished, [42] or (in other words), the new similar but stronger morbific potency controls the feelings of the patient and hence the life principle on account of its peculiarity, can no longer feel the weaker similar which becomes extinguished – exists no longer – for it was never anything material, but a dynamic – spirit-like – (conceptual) affection. The life principle henceforth is affected only and this but temporarily by the new, similar but stronger morbific potency.

§ 46

Many examples might be adduced of disease which, in the course of nature, have been homoeopathically cured by other diseases presenting similar symptoms, were it not necessary, as our object is to speak about something determinate and indubitable, to confine our attention solely to those (few) disease which are invariably the same, arise from a fixed miasm, and hence merit a distinct name.

Among these the smallpox, so dreaded on account of the great number of its serious symptoms, occupies a prominent position, and it has removed and cured a number of maladies with similar symptoms.

How frequently does smallpox produce violent ophthalmia, sometimes even causing blindness! And see! By its inoculation Dezoteux [43] cured a chronic ophthalmia permanently, and Leroy [44] another.

An amaurosis of two years' duration, consequent on suppressed scald head, was perfectly cured by it, according to Klein. [45]

How often does smallpox cause deafness and dyspnoea! And both these chronic diseases it removed on reaching its acme, as J. Fr. Closs [46] observed.

Swelling of the testicle, even of a very severe character, is a frequent symptom of small-pox, and on this account it was enabled, as Klein [47] observed, to cure, by virtue of similarity, a large hard swelling of the left testicle, consequently on a bruise. And another observer [48] saw a similar swelling of the testicle cured by it.

Among the troublesome symptoms of small-pox is a dysenteric state of the bowels; and it subdued, as Fr. Wendt [49] observed, a case of dysentery, as a similar morbific agent.

Smallpox coming on after vaccination, as well on account of its greater strength as its great similarity, at once removes entirely the cow-pox homoeopathically, and does not permit it to come to maturity; but, on the other hand, the cow-pox when near maturity does, on account of its great similarity, homoeopathically diminish very much the supervening smallpox and make it much milder [50], as Muhry [51] and many others testify.

The inoculated cow-pox, whose lymph, besides the protective matter, contains the contagion of a general cutaneous eruption of another nature, consisting of usually small, dry (rarely large, pustular) pimples, resting on a small red areola, frequently conjoined with round red cutaneous spots and often accompanied by the most violent itching, which rash appears in not a few children several days before, more frequently, however, after the red areola of the cow-pock, and goes off in a few days, leaving behind small, red, hard spots on the skin; – the inoculated cow-pox, I say, after it has taken, cures perfectly and permanently, in a homoeopathic manner, by the similarity of this accessory miasm, analogous cutaneous eruptions of children, often of very long standing and of a very troublesome character, as a number of observers assert. [52]

The cow-pox, a peculiar symptom of which is to cause tumefaction of the arm, [53] cured, after it broke out, a swollen half-paralyzed arm. [54]

The fever accompanying cow-pox, which occurs at the time of the production of the red areola, cured homoeopathically intermittent fever in two individuals, as the younger Hardege [55] reports, confirming what J. Hunter [56] had already observed, that two fevers (similar diseases) cannot co-exist in the same body.

The measles bear a strong resemblance in the character of its fever and cough to the whooping-cough, and hence it was that Bosquillon [57] noticed, in an epidemic where both these affections prevailed, that many children who then took measles remained free from whooping-cough during that epidemic. They would all have been protected from, and rendered incapable of being infected by, the whooping-cough in that and all subsequent epidemics, by the measles, if the whooping-cough were not a disease that has only a partial similarity to the measles, that is to say, if it had also a cutaneous eruption similar to what the latter possesses. As it is, however, the measles can but preserve a large number from whooping-cough homoeopathically, and that only in the epidemic prevailing at the time.

If, however, the measles come in contact with a disease resembling it in its chief symptom, the eruption, it can indisputably remove, and effect a homoeopathic cure of the latter. Thus a chronic herpetic eruption was entirely and permanently (homoeopathically) cured [58] by the breaking out of the measles, as Kortum [59] observed. An excessively burning miliary rash on the face, neck, and arms, that had lasted six years, and was aggravated by every change of weather, on the invasion of measles assumed the form of a swelling of the surface of the skin; after the measles had run its course the exanthema was cured, and returned no more. [60]

§ 47

Nothing could teach the physician in a plainer and more convincing manner than the above what kind of artificial morbific agent (medicine) he ought to choose in order to cure in a sure, rapid and permanent manner, conformably with the process that takes place in nature.

§ 48
Neither in the course of nature, as we see from all the above examples, nor by the physician's art, can an existing affection or malady in any one instance be removed by a dissimilar morbific agent, be it ever so strong, but solely by one that is similar in symptoms and is somewhat stronger, according to eternal, irrevocable laws of nature, which have not hitherto been recognized.

§ 49
We should have been able to meet with many more real, natural homoeopathic cures of this kind if, on the one hand, the attention of observers had been more directed to them, and, on the other hand, if nature had not been so deficient in helpful homoeopathic diseases.

§ 50
Mighty Nature herself has, as we see, at her command, as instruments for effecting homoeopathic cures, little besides the miasmatic diseases of constant character, (the itch) measles and smallpox [61], morbific agents which [62], as remedies, are either more dangerous to life and more to be dreaded than the disease they are to cure, they themselves require curing, in order to be eradicated in their turn – both circumstances that make their employment, as homoeopathic remedies, difficult, uncertain and dangerous. And how few diseases are there to which man is subject that find their similar remedy in smallpox, measles or itch! Hence, in the course of nature, very few maladies can be cured by these uncertain and hazardous homoeopathic remedies, and the cure by their instrumentality is also attended with danger and much difficulty, for this reason that the doses of these morbific powers cannot be diminished according to circumstances, as doses of medicine can; but the patient afflicted with an analogous malady of long standing must be subjected to the entire dangerous and tedious disease, to the entire disease of smallpox, measles (or itch), which in its turn has to be cured. And yet, as is seen, we can point to some striking homoeopathic cures effected by this lucky concurrence, all so many incontrovertible proofs of the great, the sole therapeutic law of nature that obtains in them: Cure by symptoms similarity!

§ 51
This therapeutic law is rendered obvious to all intelligent minds by these instances, and they are amply sufficient for this end. But, on the other hand, see what advantages man has over crude Nature in her happy-go-lucky operations. How many thousands more of homoeopathic morbific agents has not man at his disposal for the relief of his suffering fellow-creatures in the medicinal substances universally distributed throughout creation! In them he has producers of disease of all possible varieties of action, for all the innumerable, for all conceivable and inconceivable natural diseases, to which they can render homoeopathic aid – morbific agents (medicinal substances), whose power, when their remedial employment is completed, being overcome by the vital force, disappears spontaneously without requiring a second course of treatment for its extirpation, like the itch – artificial morbific agents, which the physician can attenuate, subdivide and potentize almost to an infinite extent, and the dose of which he can diminish to such a degree that they shall remain only slightly stronger than the similar natu-

ral disease they are employed to cure; so that in this incomparable method of cure, there is no necessity for any violent attack upon the organism for the eradication of even an inveterate disease of old standing; the cure by this method takes place by only a gentle, imperceptible and yet often rapid transition from the tormenting natural disease to the desired state of permanent health.

§ 52 Fifth Edition

Surely no intelligent physician, after these examples as clear as daylight, can still go on in the old ordinary system of medicine, attacking the body, as has hitherto been done, in its least diseased parts with (allopathic) medicines that have no direct pathological (homoeopathic) relation to the disease to be cured, with purgatives, counter-irritants, derivatives, etc. [63], and thus at a sacrifice of the patient's strength, inducing a morbid state quite heterogeneous and dissimilar to the original one, to the ruin of his constitution, by large doses of mixtures of medicines generally of unknown qualities, the employment of which can have no other result, as is demonstrated by the eternal laws of nature in the above and all other cases in the world in which a dissimilar disease is added to the other in the human organism, for a cure is never thereby effected in disease, but an aggravation is the invariable consequence, – therefore it can have no other result than that either (because, according to the process of nature described in I, the older disease in the body repels the dissimilar one wherewith the patient is assailed) the natural disease remains as it was, under mild allopathic treatment, be it ever so long continued, the patient being thereby weakened; or (because, according to the process of nature described in II, the new and stronger disease merely obscures and suspends for a short time the original weaker dissimilar one), by the violent attack on the body with strong allopathic drugs, the original disease seems to yield for a time, to return in at least all its former strength; or (because, according to the process of nature described in III, two dissimilar diseases, when both are of a chronic character and of equal strength, take up a position when beside one another in the organism and complicate each other) in those cases in which the physician employs for a long time morbific agents opposite and dissimilar to the natural chronic disease and allopathic medicines in large doses, such allopathic treatment, without ever being able to remove and to cure the original (dissimilar) chronic disease, only develops new artificial diseases beside it; and, as daily experience shows, only renders the patient much worse and more incurable than before.

§ 52 Sixth Edition

There are but two principle methods of cure: the one based only on accurate observation of nature, on careful experimentation and pure experience, the homoeopathic (before we never designedly used) and a second which does not do this, the heteropathic or allopathic. Each opposes the other, and only he who does not know either can hold the delusion that they can ever approach each other or even become united, or to make himself so ridiculous as to practice at one time homoeopathically at another allopathically, according to the pleasure of the patient; a practice which may be called criminal treason against divine homoeopathy.

§ 53 Fifth Edition

True, mild cures take place, as we see, only in a homoeopathic way – a way which, as we have also shown above (§§ 7-25) in a different manner, by experience and deductions, is also the true and only one whereby diseases may be most surely, rapidly and permanently extinguished by art; for this mode of cure is founded on an eternal, infallible law of nature.

§ 53 Sixth Edition

The true mild cures take place only according to the homoeopathic method, which, as we have found (§§ 7-25) by experience and deduction, is unquestionably the proper one by which through art the quickest, most certain and most permanent cures are obtained since this healing art rests upon an eternal infallible law of nature.

The pure homoeopathic healing art is the only correct method, the one possible to human art, the straightest way to cure, as certain as that there is but one straight line between two given points.

§ 54 Fifth Edition

This, the homoeopathic way, must, moreover, as observed above (§§ 43-49) be the only proper one, because, of the three possible modes of employing medicines in diseases, it is the only direct way to a mild, sure, permanent cure without doing injury in another direction, and without weakening the patient. The pure homoeopathic mode of cure is the only proper way, the only direct way, the only way possible to human skill, as certainly as only one straight line can be drawn betwixt two given points.

§ 54 Sixth Edition

The allopathic method of treatment utilized many things against disease, but usually only improper ones (alloea) and ruled for ages in different forms called systems. Every one of these, following each other from time to time and differing greatly each from the other, honored itself with the name of Rational Medicine. [64]

Every builder of such a system cherished the haughty estimation of himself that he was able to penetrate into the inner nature of life of the healthy as well as of the sick and clearly to recognize it and accordingly gave the prescription which noxious matter [65] should be banished from the sick man, and how to banish it in order to restore him to health, all this according to empty assumptions and arbitrary suppositions without honestly questioning nature and listening without prejudice to the voice of experience. Diseases were held to be conditions that reappeared pretty much in the same manner. Most systems gave, therefore, names to their imagined disease pictures and classified them, every system differently. To medicines were ascribed actions which were supposed to cure these abnormal conditions. (Hence the numerous text books on Materia Medica.) [66]

§ 55 Fifth Edition

The second mode of employing medicines in diseases, the allopathic or homoeopathic, which, without any pathological relation to what is actually diseased in the body, attacks the parts most exempt from the disease, in order to draw away the disease through them and thus to expel it, as is imagined, has hitherto been the most general method. I have treated of it above in the Introduction, [67] and shall not dwell longer on it.

§ 55 Sixth Edition
Soon, however, the public became convinced that the sufferings of the sick increased and heightened with the introduction of every one of these systems and methods of cure if followed exactly. Long ago these allopathic physicians would have been left had it not been for the palliative relief obtained at times from empirically discovered remedies whose almost instantaneous flattering action is apparent to the patient and this to some extent served to keep up their credit.

§ 56 Fifth Edition
The third and only remaining method [68] of employing medicines in diseases, which, besides the other two just alluded to, is the only other possible one, is the antipathic (enantiopathic) or palliative method, wherewith the physician could hitherto appear to be most useful, and hoped most certainly to gain his patient's confidence by deluding him with momentary amelioration. But I shall now proceed to show how inefficacious and how injurious this third and sole remaining way was, in diseases of a not very rapid course. It is certainly the only one of the modes of treatment adopted by the allopaths that had any manifest relation to a portion of the sufferings caused by the natural disease; but what kind of relation? Of a truth the very one (the exact contrary of the right one) that ought most to be avoided if we would not delude and make a mockery of the patient affected with a chronic disease.

§ 56 Sixth Edition
By means of this palliative (antipathic, enantiopathic) method, introduced according to Galen's teaching "Contraria contrariis" for seventeen centuries, the physicians hitherto could hope to win confidence while they deluded with almost instantaneous amelioration. But how fundamentally unhelpful and hurtful this method of treatment is (in diseases not running a rapid course) we shall see in what follows. It is certainly the only one of the modes of treatment adopted by the allopaths that had any manifest relation to a portion of the sufferings caused by the natural disease; but what kind of relation? Of a truth the very one (the exact contrary of the right one) that ought carefully to be avoided if we would not delude and make a mockery of the patient affected with a chronic disease. [69]

§ 57
In order to carry into practice this antipathic method, the ordinary physician gives, for a single troublesome symptom from among the many other symptoms of the disease which he passes by unheeded, a medicine concerning which it is known that it produces the exact opposite of the morbid symptom sought to be subdued, from which, agreeably to the fifteen – centuries – old traditional rule of the antiquated medical school (contraria contrariis) he can expect the speediest (palliative) relief. He gives large doses of opium for pains of all sorts, because this drug soon benumbs the sensibility, and administers the same remedy for diarrhoeas, because it speedily puts a stop to the peristaltic motion of the intestinal canal and makes it insensible; and also for sleeplessness, because opium rapidly produces a stupefied, comatose sleep; he gives purgatives when the patient has suffered long from constipation and costiveness; he causes the burnt hand to be plunged into cold water, which, from its low degree of temperature, seems instantaneously to remove the burning pain, as if by magic; he puts the

patient who complains of chilliness and deficiency of vital heat into warm baths, which warm him immediately; he makes him who is suffering from prolonged debility drink wine, whereby he is instantly enlivened and refreshed; and in like manner he employs other opposite (antipathic) remedial means, but he has very few besides those just mentioned, as it is only of very few substances that some peculiar (primary) action is known to the ordinary medical school.

§ 58

If, in estimating the value of this mode of employing medicines, we should even pass over the circumstance that it is an extremely faulty symptomatic treatment (v. note to § 7), wherein the practitioner devotes his attention in a merely one-sided manner to a single symptom, consequently to only a small part of the whole, whereby relief for the totality of the disease, which is what the patient desires, cannot evidently be expected, – we must, on the other hand, demand of experience if, in one single case where such antipathic employment of medicine was made use of in a chronic or persisting affection, after the transient amelioration there did not ensue an increased aggravation of the symptom which was subdued at first in a palliative manner, an aggravation, indeed, of the whole disease? And every attentive observer will agree that, after such short antipathic amelioration, aggravation follows in every case without exception, although the ordinary physician is in the habit of giving his patient another explanation of this subsequent aggravation, and ascribes it to malignancy of the original disease, now for the first time showing itself, or to the occurrence of quite a new disease. [70]

§ 59

Important symptoms of persistent diseases have never yet been treated with such palliative, antagonistic remedies, without the opposite state, a relapse – indeed, a palpable aggravation of the malady – occurring a few hours afterwards. For a persistent tendency to sleepiness during the day the physician prescribed coffee, whose primary action is to enliven; and when it had exhausted its action the day – somnolence increased; – for frequent waking at night he gave in the evening, without heeding the other symptoms of the disease, opium, which by virtue of its primary action produced the same night (stupefied, dull) sleep, but the subsequent nights were still more sleepless than before; – to chronic diarrhoeas he opposed, without regarding the other morbid signs, the same opium, whose primary action is to constipate the bowels, and after a transient stoppage of the diarrhoea it subsequently became all the worse; – violent and frequently recurring pains of all kinds he could suppress with opium for but a short time; they then always returned in greater, often intolerable severity, or some much worse affection came in their stead. For nocturnal cough of long standing the ordinary physician knew no better than to administer opium, whose primary action is to suppress every irritation; the cough would then perhaps cease the first night, but during the subsequent nights it would be still more severe, and if it were again and again suppressed by this palliative in increased doses, fever and nocturnal perspiration were added to the disease; – weakness of the bladder, with consequent retention of urine, was sought to be conquered by the antipathic work of cantharides to stimulate the urinary passages whereby evacuation of the urine was certainly at first effected but thereafter the bladder becomes less capable of stimulation and less able to contract, and paralysis of the bladder is imminent; – with large doses of purgative drugs and laxative salts, which excite the bowels to frequent evacuation, it was sought to remove a chronic tendency to constipation, but in the secondary action the bowels became still more confined; – the ordinary physician seeks to remove chronic debility by the administration of wine, which, however, stimulates only in its primary action, and hence the forces sink all the lower in the secondary its primary action, and hence the forces sink all the lower in the secondary action; – by bitter substances and heating condiments he tries to strengthen and warm the chronically weak and cold stomach, but in the secondary action of these palliatives, which are stimulating in their primary action only, the stomach becomes yet more inactive; – long standing deficiency of vital heat and chilly disposition ought surely to yield to prescriptions of warm baths, but still more weak, cold, and chilly do the patients subsequently become; – severely burnt parts feel instantaneous alleviation from the application of cold water, but the burning pain afterwards increases to an incredible degree, and the inflammation spreads and rises to a still greater height; [71] – by means of the sternutatory remedies that provoke a secretion of mucus, coryza with stoppage of the nose of long standing is sought to be removed, but it escapes observation that the disease is aggravated all the more by these antagonistic remedies (in their secondary action), and the nose becomes still more stopped; – by electricity and galvanism, with in their primary action greatly stimulate muscular action, chronically weak and almost paralytic limbs were soon excited to more active movements, but the consequence (the secondary action) was complete deadening of all muscular irritability and complete paralysis; – by venesections it was attempted to remove chronic determination of blood to the head, but they were always followed by greater congestion; – ordinary medical practitioners know nothing better with which to treat the paralytic torpor of the corporeal and mental organs, conjoined with unconsciousness, which prevails in many kinds of typhus, than with large doses of valerian, because this is one of the most powerful medicinal agents for causing animation and increasing the motor faculty; in their ignorance, however, they knew not that this action is only a primary action, and that the organism, after that is passed, most certainly falls back, in the secondary (antagonistic) action, into still greater stupor and immobility, that is to say, into paralysis of the mental and corporeal organs (and death); they did not see, that the very diseases they supplied most plentifully with valerian, which is in such cases an oppositely acting, antipathic remedy, most infallibly terminated fatally. The old school physician rejoices [72] that he is able to reduce for several hours the velocity of the small rapid pulse in cachectic patients with the very first dose of uncombined purple foxglove (which in its primary action makes the pulse slower); its rapidity, however, soon returns; repeated, and now increased doses effect an ever smaller diminution of its rapidity, and at length none at all – indeed – in the secondary action the pulse becomes uncountable; sleep, appetite and strength depart, and a speedy death is invariably the result, or else insanity ensues. How often, in one word, the disease is aggravated, or something even worse is effected by the secondary action of such antagonistic (antipathic) remedies, the old school with its false theories does not perceive, but experience teaches it in a terrible manner.

§ 60 Fifth Edition
If these ill-effects are produced, as may very naturally be expected from the antipathic employment of medicines, the ordinary physician imagines he can get over the difficulty by giving, at each renewed aggravation, a stronger dose of the remedy, whereby an equally transient suppression is effected; and as there then is a still greater necessity for giving ever-increasing quantities of the palliative there ensues either another more serious disease or frequently even danger to life and death itself, but never a cure of a disease of considerable or of long standing.

§ 60 Sixth Edition
If these ill-effects are produced, as may very naturally be expected from the antipathic employment of medicines, the ordinary physician imagines he can get over the difficulty by giving, at each renewed aggravation, a stronger dose of the remedy, whereby an equally transient suppression [73] is effected; and as there then is a still greater necessity for giving ever – increasing quantities of the palliative there ensues either another more serious disease or frequently even danger to life and death itself, but never a cure of a disease of considerable or of long standing.

§ 61
Had physicians been capable of reflecting on the sad results of the antagonistic employment of medicines, they had long since discovered the grand truth, THAT THE TRUE RADICAL HEALING ART MUST BE FOUND IN THE EXACT OPPOSITE OF SUCH AN ANTIPATHIC TREATMENT OF THE SYMPTOMS OF DISEASE; they would have become convinced, that as a medicinal action antagonistic to the symptoms of the disease (an antipathically employed medicine) is followed by only transient relief, and after that is passed, by invariable aggravation, the converse of that procedure, the homoeopathic employment of medicines according to similarity of symptoms, must effect a permanent and perfect cure, if at the same time the opposite of their large doses, the most minute doses, are exhibited. But neither the obvious aggravation that ensued from their antipathic treatment, nor the fact that no physician ever effected a permanent cure of disease of considerable or of long standing unless some homoeopathic medicinal agent was accidentally a chief ingredient in his prescription, nor yet the circumstances that all the rapid and perfect cures that nature ever performed (§ 46), were always effected by the supervention upon the old disease of one of a similar character, ever taught them, during such a long series of centuries, this truth, the knowledge of which can alone conduce to the benefit of the sick.

§ 62
But on what this pernicious result of the palliative, antipathic treatment and the efficacy of the reverse, the homoeopathic treatment, depend, is explained by the following facts, deduced from manifold observations, which no one before me perceived, though they are so very palpable and so very evident, and are of such infinite importance to the healing art.

§ 63
Every agent that acts upon the vitality, every medicine, deranges more or less the vital force, and causes a certain alteration in the health of the individual for a

longer or a shorter period. This is termed primary action. Although a product of the medicinal and vital powers conjointly, it is principally due to the former power. To its action our vital force endeavors to oppose its own energy. This resistant action is a property, is indeed an automatic action of our life-preserving power, which goes by the name of secondary action or counteraction.

§ 64

During the primary action of the artificial morbific agents (medicines) on our healthy body, as seen in the following examples, our vital force seems to conduct itself merely in a passive (receptive) manners, and appears, so to say, compelled to permit the impressions of the artificial power acting from without to take place in it and thereby after its state of health; it then, however, appears to rouse itself again, as it were, and to develop (A) the exact opposite condition of health (counteraction, secondary action) to this effect (primary action) produced upon it, if there be such an opposite, and that in as great a degree as was the effect (primary action) of the artificial morbific agent on it, and proportionate to its own energy; – or (B) if there be not in nature a state exactly the opposite of the primary action, it appears to endeavor to indifferentiate itself, that is, to make its superior power available in the extinction of the change wrought in it from without (by the medicine), in the place of which it substitutes its normal state (secondary action, curative action).

§ 65

Examples of (A) are familiar to all. A hand bathed in hot water is at first much warmer than the other hand that has not been so treated (primary action); but when it is withdrawn from the hot water and again thoroughly dried, it becomes in a short time cold, and at length much colder than the other (secondary action). A person heated by violent exercise (primary action) is afterwards affected with chilliness and shivering (secondary action). To one who was yesterday heated by drinking much wine (primary action), today every breath of air feels too cold (counteraction of the organism, secondary action). An arm that has been kept long in very cold water is at first much paler and colder (primary action) than the other; but removed from the cold water and dried, it subsequently becomes not only warmer than the other, but even hot, red and inflamed (secondary action, reaction of the vital force). Excessive vivacity follows the use of strong coffee (primary action), but sluggishness and drowsiness remain for a long time afterwards (reaction, secondary action), if this be not always again removed for a short time by imbibing fresh supplies of coffee (palliative). After the profound stupefied sleep caused by opium (primary action), the following night will be all the more sleepless (reaction, secondary action). After the constipation produced by opium (primary action), diarrhoea ensues (secondary action); and after purgation with medicines that irritate the bowels, constipation of several days' duration ensues (secondary action). And in like manner it always happens, after the primary action of a medicine that produces in large doses a great change in the health of a healthy person, that its exact opposite, when, as has been observed, there is actually such a thing, is produced in the secondary action by our vital force.

§ 66

An obvious antagonistic secondary action, however, is, as may readily be conceived, not to be noticed from the action of quite minute homoeopathic doses of the deranging agents on the healthy body. A small dose of every one of them certainly produces a primary action that is perceptible to a sufficiently attentive; but the living organism employs against it only so much reaction (secondary action) as is necessary for the restoration of the normal condition.

§ 67 Fifth Edition
These incontrovertible truths, which spontaneously offer themselves to our notice and experience, explain to us the beneficial action that takes place under homoeopathic treatment; while, on the other hand, they demonstrate the perversity of the antipathic and palliative treatment of diseases with antagonistically acting medicines. [74]

§ 67 Sixth Edition
These incontrovertible truths, which spontaneously offer themselves to our notice and experience, explain to us the beneficial action that takes place under homoeopathic treatment; while, on the other hand, they demonstrate the perversity of the antipathic and palliative treatment of diseases with antagonistically acting medicines. [74]

§ 68 Fifth Edition
In homoeopathic cures they show us that from the uncommonly small doses of medicine (§§ 275 – 287) required in this method of treatment, which are just sufficient, by the similarity of their symptoms, to overpower and remove the similar nature disease, there certainly remains, after the destruction of the latter, at first a certain amount of medicinal disease alone in the organism, but, on account of the extraordinary minuteness of the dose, it is so transient, so slight, and disappears so rapidly of its own accord, that the vital force has no need to employ, against this small artificial derangement of its health, any more considerable reaction than will suffice to elevate its present state of health up to the healthy point – that is, than will suffice to effect complete recovery, for which after the extinction of the previous morbid derangement but little effort is required (§ 64, B).

§ 68 Sixth Edition
In homoeopathic cures they show us that from the uncommonly small doses of medicine (§§ 275 – 287) required in this method of treatment, which are just sufficient, by the similarity of their symptoms, to overpower and remove from the sensation of the life principle the similar natural disease there certainly remains, after the destruction of the latter, at first a certain amount of medicinal disease alone in the organism, but, on account of the extraordinary minuteness of the dose, it is so transient, so slight, and disappears so rapidly of its own accord, that the vital force has no need to employ, against this small artificial derangement of its health, any more considerable reaction than will suffice to elevate its present state of health up to the healthy point – that is, than will suffice to effect complete recovery, for which after the extinction of the previous morbid derangement but little effort is required (§ 64, B).

§ 69 Fifth Edition
In the antipathic (palliative) mode of treatment, however precisely the reverse of this takes place. The medicinal symptom which the physician opposes to the dis-

ease symptom (for example, the insensibility and stupefaction caused by opium in its primary action to acute pain) is certainly not alien, not allopathic of the latter; there is a manifest relation of the medicinal symptom to the disease symptom, but it is the reverse of what should be; it is here intended that the annihilation of the disease symptom shall be effected by an opposite medicinal symptom, which is impossible. No doubt the antipathically chosen medicine touches precisely the same diseased point in the organism as the homoeopathic medicine chosen on account of the similar affection it produces; but the former covers the opposite symptom of the disease only as an opposite, and makes it unobservable for a short time only, so that in the first period of the action of the antagonistic palliative the vital force perceives nothing disagreeable from either if the two (neither from the disease symptom nor from the medicinal symptom), as they seem both to have mutually removed and dynamically neutralized one another as it were (for example, the stupefying power of opium does this to the pain). In the first minutes the vital force feels quite well, and perceives neither the stupefaction of the opium nor the pain of the disease. But as the antagonistic medicinal symptom cannot (as in the homoeopathic treatment) occupy the place of the morbid derangement present in the organism as a similar, stronger (artificial) disease, and cannot, therefore, like a homoeopathic medicine, affect the vital force with a similar artificial disease, so as to be able to step into the place of the original natural morbid derangement, the palliative medicine must, as a thing totally differing from, and the opposite of the disease derangement, leave the latter uneradicated; it renders it, as before said, by a semblance of dynamic neutralization, [75] at first unfelt by the vital force, but, like every medicinal disease, it is soon spontaneously extinguished, and not only leaves the disease behind, just as it was, but compels the vital force (as it must, like all palliatives, be given in large doses in order to effect the apparent removal) to produce an opposite condition (§§ 63,64) to this palliative medicine, the reverse of the medicinal action, consequently the analogue of the still present, undestroyed, natural morbid derangement, which is necessarily strengthened and increased [76] by this addition (reaction against the palliative) produced by the vital force. The disease symptom (this single part of the disease) consequently becomes worse after the term of the action of the palliative has expired; worse in proportion to the magnitude of the dose of the palliative. Accordingly (to keep to the same example) the larger the dose of opium given to allay the pain, so much the more does the pain increase beyond its original intensity as soon as the opium has exhausted its action. [77]

§ 69 Sixth Edition

In the antipathic (palliative) mode of treatment, however precisely the reverse of this takes place. The medicinal symptom which the physician opposes to the disease symptom (for example, the insensibility and stupefaction caused by opium in its primary action to acute pain) is certainly not alien, not allopathic of the latter; there is a manifest relation of the medicinal symptom to the disease symptom, but it is the reverse of what should be; it is here intended that the annihilation of the disease symptom shall be effected by an opposite medicinal symptom, which is nevertheless impossible. No doubt the antipathically chosen medicine touches precisely the same diseased point in the organism as the homoeopathic medicine chosen on account of the similar affection it produces; but the former covers the opposite symptom of the disease only as an opposite, and makes it unobservable to our life principle for a short time only, so that in the first period of the action of the antagonistic palliative the vital force perceives nothing disagreeable from either if the two (neither from the disease symptom nor from the medicinal symptom), as they seem both to have mutually removed and dynamically neutralized one another as it were (for example, the stupefying power of opium does this to the pain). In the first minutes the vital force feels quite well, and perceives neither the stupefaction of the opium nor the pain of the disease. But as the antagonistic medicinal symptom cannot (as in the homoeopathic treatment) occupy the place of the morbid derangement present in the organism in the sensation of the life principle as a similar, stronger (artificial) disease, and cannot, therefore, like a homoeopathic medicine, affect the vital force with a similar artificial disease, so as to be able to step into the place of the original natural morbid derangement, the palliative medicine must, as a thing totally differing from, and the opposite of the disease derangement, leave the latter uneradicated; it renders it, as before said, by a semblance of dynamic neutralization, [75] at first unfelt by the vital force, but, like every medicinal disease, it is soon spontaneously extinguished, and not only leaves the disease behind, just as it was, but compels the vital force (as it must, like all palliatives, be given in large doses in order to effect the apparent removal) to produce an opposite condition (§§ 63,64) to this palliative medicine, the reverse of the medicinal action, consequently the analogue of the still present, undestroyed, natural morbid derangement, which is necessarily strengthened and increased [76] by this addition (reaction against the palliative) produced by the vital force. The disease symptom (this single part of the disease) consequently becomes worse after the term of the action of the palliative has expired; worse in proportion to the magnitude of the dose of the palliative. Accordingly (to keep to the same example) the larger the dose of opium given to allay the pain, so much the more does the pain increase beyond its original intensity as soon as the opium has exhausted its action. [77]

§ 70 Fifth Edition
From what has been already adduced we cannot fail to draw the following inferences:

That everything of a really morbid character and which ought to be cured that the physician can discover in diseases consists solely of the sufferings of the patient, and the sensible alterations in his health, in a word, solely of the totality of the symptoms, by means of which the disease demands the medicine requisite for its relief; while, on the other hand, every internal cause attributed to it, every occult quality or imaginary material morbific principle, is nothing but an idle dream;

That this derangement of the state of health, which we term disease, can only be converted into health by another revolution effected in the state of health by means of medicines, whose sole curative power, consequently, can only consist in altering man's state of health – that is to say, in a peculiar excitation of morbid symptoms, and is learned with most distinctness and purity by testing them on the healthy body;

That, according to all experience, a natural disease can never be cured by medicines that possess the power of producing in the healthy individual an alien morbid state (dissimilar morbid symptoms) differing from that of the disease to be cured (never, therefore, by an allopathic mode of treatment), and that even in nature no cure ever takes place in which an inherent disease is removed, annihilated and cured by the addition of another disease dissimilar to it, be the new one ever so strong;

That, moreover, all experience proves that, by means of medicines which have a tendency to produce in the healthy individual an artificial morbid symptom, antagonistic to the single symptom of disease sought to be cured, the cure of a long-standing affection will never be effected, but merely a very transientalleviation, always follows by its aggravation; and that, in a word, this antipathic and merely palliative treatment in long-standing diseases of a serious character is absolutely inefficacious;

That, however, the third and only other possible mode of treatment (the homoeopathic), in which there is employed for the totality of the symptoms of a natural disease a medicine capable of producing the most similar symptoms possible in the healthy individual, given in suitable dose, is the only efficacious remedial method whereby diseases, which are purely dynamic deranging irritations of the vital force, are overpowered, and being thus easily, perfectly and permanently extinguished, must necessarily cease to exist – and for this mode of procedure we have the example of unfettered Nature herself, when to an old disease there is added a new one similar to the first, whereby the new one is rapidly and forever annihilated and cured.

§ 70 Sixth Edition

From what has been already adduced we cannot fail to draw the following inferences:

That everything of a really morbid character and which ought to be cured that the physician can discover in diseases consists solely of the sufferings of the patient, and the sensible alterations in his health, in a word, solely of the totality of the symptoms, by means of which the disease demands the medicine requisite for its relief; while, on the other hand, every internal cause attributed to it, every occult quality or imaginary material morbific principle, is nothing but an idle dream;

That this derangement of the state of health, which we term disease, can only be converted into health by another revolution effected in the state of health by means of medicines, whose sole curative power, consequently, can only consist in altering man's state of health – that is to say, in a peculiar excitation of morbid symptoms, and is learned with most distinctness and purity by testing them on the healthy body;

That, according to all experience, a natural disease can never be cured by medicines that possess the power of producing in the healthy individual an alien morbid state (dissimilar morbid symptoms) differing from that of the disease to be cured (never, therefore, by an allopathic mode of treatment), and that even in nature no cure ever takes place in which an inherent disease is removed, annihilated and cured by the addition of another disease dissimilar to it, be the new one ever so strong;

That, moreover, all experience proves that, by means of medicines which have a tendency to produce in the healthy individual an artificial morbid symptom, antagonistic to the single symptom of disease sought to be cured, the cure of a long-standing affection will never be effected, but merely a very transientallevia-tion, always follows by its aggravation; and that, in a word, this antipathic and merely palliative treatment in long-standing diseases of a serious character is absolutely inefficacious;

That, however, the third and only other possible mode of treatment (the homoeopathic), in which there is employed for the totality of the symptoms of a natural disease a medicine capable of producing the most similar symptoms possible in the healthy individual, given in suitable dose, is the only efficacious remedial method whereby diseases, which are purely dynamic deranging irritations of the vital force, are overpowered, and being thus easily, perfectly and permanently extinguished, must necessarily cease to exist. This is brought about by means of the stronger similar deranging irritation of the homoeopathic medicine in the sensation of the life principle. – and for this mode of procedure we have the example of unfettered Nature herself, when to an old disease there is added a new one similar to the first, whereby the new one is rapidly and forever annihilated and cured.

§ 71

As it is now no longer a matter of doubt that the diseases of mankind consist merely of groups of certain symptoms, and may be annihilated and transformed into health by medicinal substances, but only by such as are capable of artificially producing similar morbid symptoms (and such is the process in all genuine cures), hence the operation of curing is comprised in the three following points:

I. How is the physician to ascertain what is necessary to be known in order to cure the disease?

II. How is he to gain a knowledge of the instruments adapted for the cure of the natural disease, the pathogenetic powers of the medicines?

III. What is the most suitable method of employing these artificial morbific agents (medicines) for the cure of natural disease?

§ 72

With respect to the first point, the following will serve as a general preliminary view. The disease to which man is liable are either rapid morbid processes of the abnormally deranged vital force, which have a tendency to finish their course more or less quickly, but always in a moderate time – these are termed acute diseases; – or they are diseases of such a character that, with small, often imperceptible beginnings, dynamically derange the living organism, each in its own peculiar manner, and cause it gradually to deviate from the healthy condition, in such a way that the automatic life energy, called vital force, whose office is to preserve the health, only opposes to them at the commencement and during their progress imperfect, unsuitable, useless resistance, but is unable of itself to extinguish them, but must helplessly suffer (them to spread and) itself to be ever more and more abnormally deranged, until at length the organism is destroyed; these are termed chronic diseases. They are caused by infection with a chronic miasm.

§ 73

As regards acute diseases, they are either of such a kind as attack human beings individually, the exciting cause being injurious influences to which they were particularly exposed. Excesses in food, or an insufficient supply of it, severe physical impression, chills, over heatings, dissipation, strains, etc., or physical irritations, mental emotions, and the like, are exciting causes of such acute febrile affections; in reality, however, they are generally only a transient explosion of latent psora, which spontaneously returns to its dormant state if the acute diseases were not of too violent a character and were soon quelled. Or they are of such a kind as attack several persons at the same time, here and there (sporadically), by means of meteoric or telluric influences and injurious agents, the susceptibility for being morbidly affected by which is possessed by only a few persons at one time. Allied to these are those diseases in which many persons are attacked with very similar sufferings from the same cause (epidemically); these diseases generally become infectious (contagious) when they prevail among thickly congregated masses of human beings. Thence arise fevers [78], in each instance of a peculiar nature, and, because the cases of disease have an identical origin, they set up in all those they affect an identical morbid process, which when left to itself terminates in a moderate period of time in death or recovery. The calamities of war, inundations and famine are not infrequently their exciting causes and producers – sometimes they are peculiar acute miasms which recur in the same manner (hence known by some traditional name), which either attack persons but once in a lifetime, as the smallpox, measles, whooping-cough, the ancient, smooth, bright red scarlet fever [79] of Sydenham, the mumps, etc., or such as recur frequently in pretty much the same manner, the plague of the Levant, the yellow fever of the sea-coast, the Asiatic cholera, etc.

§ 74 Fifth Edition

Among chronic diseases we must still, alas!, reckon those so commonly met with, artificially produced in allopathic treatment by the prolonged use of violent heroic medicines in large and increasing doses, by the abuse of calomel, corrosive sublimate, mercurial ointment, nitrate of silver, iodine and its ointments, opium, valerian, cinchona bark and quinine, foxglove, prussic acid, sulphur and sulphuric acid, perennial purgatives, venesections, leeches, issues, setons, etc., whereby the vital force is sometimes weakened to an unmerciful extent, sometimes, if it do not succumb, gradually abnormally deranged (by each substance in a peculiar manner) in such a way that, in order to maintain life against these inimical and destructive attacks, it must produce a revolution in the organism, and either deprive some part of its irritability and sensibility, or exalt these to an excessive degree, cause dilatation or contraction, relaxation or induration or even total destruction of certain parts, and develop faulty organic alterations here and there in the interior or the exterior [80] (cripple the body internally or externally), in order to preserve the organism from complete destruction of the life by the ever-renewed, hostile assaults of such destructive forces.

§ 74 Sixth Edition

Among chronic diseases we must still, alas!, reckon those so commonly met with, artificially produced in allopathic treatment by the prolonged use of violent heroic medicines in large and increasing doses, by the abuse of calomel, corrosive sublimate, mercurial ointment, nitrate of silver, iodine and its ointments, opium, valerian, cinchona bark and quinine, foxglove, prussic acid, sulphur and sulphuric acid, perennial purgatives [81], venesections, shedding streams of blood, leeches, issues, setons, etc., whereby the vital energy is sometimes weakened to an unmerciful extent, sometimes, if it do not succumb, gradually abnormally deranged (by each substance in a peculiar manner) in such a way that, in order to maintain life against these inimical and destructive attacks, it must produce a revolution in the organism, and either deprive some part of its irritability and sensibility, or exalt these to an excessive degree, cause dilatation or contraction, relaxation or induration or even total destruction of certain parts, and develop faulty organic alterations here and there in the interior or the exterior (cripple the body internally or externally), in order to preserve the organism from complete destruction of the life by the ever – renewed, hostile assaults of such destructive forces. [82]

§ 75
These inroads on human health effected by the allopathic non-healing art (more particularly in recent times) are of all chronic diseases the most deplorable, the most incurable; and I regret to add that it is apparently impossible to discover or to hit upon any remedies for their cure when they have reached any considerable height.

§ 76 Fifth Edition
Only for natural diseases has the beneficent Deity granted us, in Homoeopathy, the means of affording relief; but those devastations and maimings of the human organism exteriorly and interiorly, effected by years, frequently, of the unsparing exercise of a false art, with its hurtful drugs and treatment, must be remedied by the vital force itself (appropriate aid being given for the eradication of any chronic miasm that may happen to be lurking in the background), if it has not already been too much weakened by such mischievous acts, and can devote several years to this huge operation undisturbed. A human healing art, for the restoration to the normal state of those innumerable abnormal conditions so often produced by the allopathic non-healing art, there is not and cannot be.

§ 76 Sixth Edition
Only for natural diseases has the beneficent Deity granted us, in Homoeopathy, the means of affording relief; but those devastations and maimings of the human organism exteriorly and interiorly, effected by years, frequently, of the unsparing exercise of a false art, [83] with its hurtful drugs and treatment, must be remedied by the vital force itself (appropriate aid being given for the eradication of any chronic miasm that may happen to be lurking in the background), if it has not already been too much weakened by such mischievous acts, and can devote several years to this huge operation undisturbed. A human healing art, for the restoration to the normal state of those innumerable abnormal conditions so often produced by the allopathic non-healing art, there is not and cannot be.

§ 77
Those diseases are inappropriately named chronic, which persons incur who expose themselves continually to avoidable noxious influences, who are in the habit of indulging in injurious liquors or aliments, are addicted to dissipation of many kinds which undermine the health, who undergo prolonged abstinence from things that are necessary for the support of life, who reside in unhealthy

localities, especially marshy districts, who are housed in cellars or other confined dwellings, who are deprived of exercise or of open air, who ruin their health by overexertion of body or mind, who live in a constant state of worry, etc. These states of ill-health, which persons bring upon themselves, disappear spontaneously, provided no chronic miasm lurks in the body, under an improved mode of living, and they cannot be called chronic diseases.

§ 78 Fifth Edition

The true natural chronic diseases are those that arise from a chronic miasm, which when left to themselves, and unchecked by the employment of those remedies that are specific for them, always go on increasing and growing worse, notwithstanding the best mental and corporeal regimen, and torment the patient to the end of his life with ever aggravated sufferings. These are the most numerous and greatest scourges of the human race; for the most robust constitution, the best regulated mode of living and the most vigorous energy of the vital force are insufficient for their eradication.

§ 78 Sixth Edition

The true natural chronic diseases are those that arise from a chronic miasm, which when left to themselves, and unchecked by the employment of those remedies that are specific for them, always go on increasing and growing worse, notwithstanding the best mental and corporeal regimen, and torment the patient to the end of his life with ever aggravated sufferings. These, excepting those produced by medical malpractice (§ 74), are the most numerous and greatest scourges of the human race; for the most robust constitution, the best regulated mode of living and the most vigorous energy of the vital force are insufficient for their eradication. [84]

§ 79

Hitherto syphilis alone has been to some extent known as such a chronic miasmatic disease, which when uncured ceases only with the termination of life. Sycosis (the condylomatous disease), equally ineradicable by the vital force without proper medicinal treatment, was not recognized as a chronic miasmatic disease of a peculiar character, which it nevertheless undoubtedly is, and physicians imagined they had cured it when they had destroyed the growths upon the skin, but the persisting dyscrasia occasioned by it escaped their observation.

§ 80

Incalculably greater and more important than the two chronic miasms just named, however, is the chronic miasm of psora, which, while those two reveal their specific internal dyscrasia, the one by the venereal chancre, the other by the cauliflower-like growths, does also, after the completion of the internal infection of the whole organism, announce by a peculiar cutaneous eruption, sometimes consisting only of a few vesicles accompanied by intolerable voluptuous tickling itching (and a peculiar odor), the monstrous internal chronic miasm – the psora, the only real fundamental cause and producer of all the other numerous, I may say innumerable, forms of disease, [85] which, under the names of nervous debility, hysteria, hypochondriasis, mania, melancholia, imbecility, madness, epilepsy and convulsions of all sorts, softening of the bones (rachitis), scoliosis and cyphosis, caries, cancer, fungus nematodes, neoplasms, gout, haemorrhoids, jaundice, cyanosis, dropsy, amenorrhoea, haemorrhage from the stomach, nose, lungs, bladder and womb, of asthma and ulceration of the lungs, of impotence and barrenness, of megrim, deafness, cataract, amaurosis, urinary calculus, paralysis, defects of the senses and pains of thousands of kinds, etc., figure in systematic works on pathology as peculiar, independent diseases.

§ 81
The fact that this extremely ancient infecting agent has gradually passed, in some hundreds of generations, through many millions of human organisms and has thus attained an incredible development, renders it in some measure conceivable how it can now display such innumerable morbid forms in the great family of mankind, particularly when we consider what a number of circumstances [86] contribute to the production of these great varieties of chronic diseases (secondary symptoms of psora), besides the indescribable diversity of men in respect of their congenital corporeal constitutions, so that it is no wonder if such a variety of injurious agencies, acting from within and from without and sometimes continually, on such a variety of organisms permeated with the psoric miasm, should produce an innumerable variety of defects, injuries, derangements and sufferings, which have hitherto been treated of in the old pathological works, [87] under a number of special names, as diseases of an independent character.

§ 82
Although, by the discovery of that great source of chronic diseases, as also by the discovery of the specific homoeopathic remedies for the psora, medicine has advanced some steps nearer to a knowledge of the nature of the majority of diseases it has to cure, yet, for settling the indication in each case of chronic (psoric) disease he is called on to cure, the duty of a careful apprehension of its ascertainable symptoms and characteristics is as indispensable for the homoeopathic physician as it was before that discovery, as no real cure of this or of other diseases can take place without a strict particular treatment (individualization) of each case of disease – only that in this investigation some difference is to be made when the affection is an acute and rapidly developed disease, and when it is a chronic one; seeing that, in acute disease, the chief symptoms strike us and become evident to the senses more quickly, and hence much less time is requisite for tracing the picture of the disease and much fewer questions are required to be asked1, as almost everything is self-evident, than in a chronic disease which has been gradually progressing for several years, in which the symptoms are much more difficult to be ascertained.

§ 83
This individualizing examination of a case of disease, for which I shall only give in this place general directions, of which the practitioner will bear in mind only what is applicable for each individual case, demands of the physician nothing but freedom from prejudice and sound senses, attention in observing and fidelity in tracing the picture of the disease.

§ 84
The patient details the history of his sufferings; those about him tell what they heard him complain of, how he has behaved and what they have noticed in him; the physician sees, hears, and remarks by his other senses what there is of an altered or unusual character about him. He writes down accurately all that the patient and his friends have told him in the very expressions used by them.

Keeping silence himself he allows them to say all they have to say, and refrains from interrupting them [89] unless they wander off to other matters. The physician advises them at the beginning of the examination to speak slowly, in order that he may take down in writing the important parts of what the speakers say.

§ 85

He begins a fresh line with every new circumstance mentioned by the patient or his friends, so that the symptoms shall be all ranged separately one below the other. He can thus add to any one, that may at first have been related in too vague a manner, but subsequently more explicitly explained.

§ 86

When the narrators have finished what they would say of their own accord, the physician then reverts to each particular symptom and elicits more precise information respecting it in the following manner; he reads over the symptoms as they were related to him one by one, and about each of them he inquires for further particulars, e.g., at what period did this symptom occur? Was it previous to taking the medicine he had hitherto been using? While taking the medicine? Or only some days after leaving off the medicine? What kind of pain, what sensation exactly, was it that occurred on this spot? Where was the precise spot? Did the pain occur in fits and by itself, at various times? Or was it continued, without intermission? How long did it last? At what time of the day or night, and in what position of the body was it worst, or ceased entirely? What was the exact nature of this or that event or circumstance mentioned – described in plain words?

§ 87

And thus the physician obtains more precise information respecting each particular detail, but without ever framing his questions so as to suggest the answer to the patient, [90] so that he shall only have to answer yes or no; else he will be misled to answer in the affirmative or negative something untrue, half true, or not strictly correct, either from indolence or in order to please his interrogator, from which a false picture of the disease and an unsuitable mode of treatment must result.

§ 88

If in these voluntary details nothing has been mentioned respecting several parts or functions of the body or his metal state, the physician asks what more can be told in regard to these parts and these functions, or the state of his disposition or mind, [91] but in doing this he only makes use of general expressions, in order that his informants may be obliged to enter into special details concerning them.

§ 89

When the patient (for it is on him we have chiefly to rely for a description of his sensations, except in the case of feigned diseases) has by these details, given of his own accord and in answer to inquiries, furnished the requisite information and traced a tolerably perfect picture of the disease, the physician is at liberty and obliged (if he feels he has not yet gained all the information he needs) to ask more precise, more special questions. [92]

§ 90

When the physician has finished writing down these particulars, he then makes a note of what he himself observes in the patient, [93] and ascertains how much of that was peculiar to the patient in his healthy state.

§ 91

The symptoms and feelings of the patient during a previous course of medicine do not furnish the pure picture of the disease; but on the other hand, those symptoms and ailments which he suffered from before the use of the medicines, or after they had been discontinued for several days, give the true fundamental idea of the original form of the disease, and these especially the physician must take note of. When the disease is of a chronic character, and the patient has been taking medicine up to the time he is seen, the physician may with advantage leave him some days quite without medicine, or in the meantime administer something of an unmedicinal nature and defer to a subsequent period the more precise scrutiny of the morbid symptoms, in order to be able to grasp in their purity the permanent uncontaminated symptoms of the old affection and to form a faithful picture of the disease.

§ 92

But if it be a disease of a rapid course, and if its serious character admit of no delay, the physician must content himself with observing the morbid condition, altered though it may be by medicines, if he cannot ascertain what symptoms were present before the employment of the medicines, – in order that he may at least form a just apprehension of the complete picture of the disease in its actual condition, that is to say, of the conjoint malady formed by the medicinal and original diseases, which from the use of inappropriate drugs is generally more serious and dangerous than was the original disease, and hence demands prompt and efficient aid; and by thus tracing out the complete picture of the disease he will be enabled to combat it with a suitable homoeopathic remedy, so that the patient shall not fall a sacrifice to the injurious drugs he was swallowed.

§ 93

If the disease has been brought on a short time or, in the case of a chronic affection, a considerable time previously, by some obvious cause, then the patient – or his friends when questioned privately – will mention it either spontaneously or when carefully interrogated. [94]

§ 94

While inquiring into the state of chronic disease, the particular circumstances of the patient with regard to his ordinary occupations, his usual mode of living and diet, his domestic situation, and so forth, must be well considered and scrutinized, to ascertain what there is in them that may tend to produce or to maintain disease, in order that by their removal the recovery may by prompted. [95]

§ 95

In chronic disease the investigation of the signs of disease above mentioned, and of all others, must be pursued as carefully and circumstantially as possible, and the most minute peculiarities must be attended to, partly because in these diseases they are the most characteristic and least resemble those of acute diseases, and if a cure is to be affected they cannot be too accurately noted; partly because the patients become so used to their long sufferings that they pay little or no heed to the lesser accessory symptoms, which are often very pregnant with meaning (characteristic) – often very useful in determining the choice of the remedy – and regard them almost as a necessary part of their condition, almost as health, the real feeling of which they have well-nigh forgotten in the sometimes fifteen or twenty years of suffering, and they can scarcely bring themselves to believe that these accessory symptoms, these greater or less deviations from the healthy state, can have any connection with their principal malady.

§ 96
Besides this, patients themselves differ so much in their dispositions, that some, especially the so-called hypochondriacs and other persons of great sensitiveness and impatient of suffering, portray their symptoms in too vivid colors and, in order to induce the physician to give them relief, describe their ailments in exaggerated expression. [96]

§ 97
Other individuals of an opposite character, however, partly from indolence, partly from false modesty, partly from a kind of mildness of disposition or weakness of mind, refrain from mentioning a number of their symptoms, describe them in vague terms, or allege some of them to be of no consequence.

§ 98
Now, as certainly as we should listen particularly to the patient's description of his sufferings and sensations, and attach credence especially to his own expressions wherewith he endeavors to make us understand his ailments – because in the mouths of his friends and attendants they are usually altered and erroneously stated, – so certainly, on the other hand, in all diseases, but especially in the chronic ones, the investigation of the true, complete picture and its peculiarities demands especial circumspection, tact, knowledge of human nature, caution in conducting the inquiry and patience in an eminent degree.

§ 99
On the whole, the investigation of acute diseases, or of such as have existed but a short time, is much the easiest for the physician, because all the phenomena and deviations from the health that has been put recently lost are still fresh in the memory of the patient and his friends, still continue to be novel and striking. The physician certainly requires to know everything in such cases also; but he has much less to inquire into; they are for the most part spontaneously detailed to him.

§ 100
In investigating the totality of the symptoms of epidemic and sporadic diseases it is quite immaterial whether or not something similar has ever appeared in the world before under the same or any other name. The novelty or peculiarity of a disease of that kind makes no difference either in the mode of examining or of treating it, as the physician must any way regard to pure picture of every prevailing disease as if it were something new and unknown, and investigate it thoroughly for itself, if he desire to practice medicine in a real and radical manner, never substituting conjecture for actual observation, never taking for granted that the case of disease before him is already wholly or partially known, but always carefully examining it in all its phases; and this mode of procedure is all the more requisite in such cases, as a careful examination will show that every prevailing disease is in many respects a phenomenon of a unique character, differing vastly from all previous epidemics, to which certain names have been falsely applied – with the exception of those epidemics resulting from a contagious principle that always remains the same, such as smallpox, measles, etc.

§ 101

It may easily happen that in the first case of an epidemic disease that presents itself to the physician's notice he does not at once obtain a knowledge of its complete picture, as it is only by a close observation of several cases of every such collective disease that he can become conversant with the totality of its signs and symptoms. The carefully observing physician can, however, from the examination of even the first and second patients, often arrive so nearly at a knowledge of the true state as to have in his mind a characteristic portrait of it, and even to succeed in finding a suitable, homoeopathically adapted remedy for it.

§ 102

In the course of writing down the symptoms of several cases of this kind the sketch of the disease picture becomes ever more and more complete, not more spun out and verbose, but more significant (more characteristic), and including more of the peculiarities of this collective disease; on the one hand, the general symptoms (e.g., loss of appetite, sleeplessness, etc.) become precisely defined as to their peculiarities; and on the other, the more marked and special symptoms which are peculiar to but few diseases and of rarer occurrence, at least in the same combination, become prominent and constitute what is characteristic of this malady. [97] All those affected with the disease prevailing at a given time have certainly contracted it from one and the same source and hence are suffering from the same disease; but the whole extent of such an epidemic disease and the totality of its symptoms (the knowledge whereof, which is essential for enabling us to choose the most suitable homoeopathic remedy for this array of symptoms, is obtained by a complete survey of the morbid picture) cannot be learned from one single patient, but is only to be perfectly deduced (abstracted) and ascertained from the sufferings of several patients of different constitutions.

§ 103

In the same manner as has here been taught relative to the epidemic disease, which are generally of an acute character, the miasmatic chronic maladies, which, as I have shown, always remain the same in their essential nature, especially the psora, must be investigated, as to the whole sphere of their symptoms, in a much more minute manner than has ever been done before, for in them also one patient only exhibits a portion of their symptoms, a second, a third, and so on, present some other symptoms, which also are but a (dissevered, as it were), portion of the totality of the symptoms which constitute the entire extent of this malady, so that the whole array of the symptoms belonging to such a miasmatic, chronic disease, and especially to the psora, can only be ascertained from the observation of very many single patients affected with such a chronic disease, and without a complete survey and collective picture of these symptoms the medicines capable of curing the whole malady homoeopathically (to wit, the antipsorics) cannot be discovered; and these medicines are, at the same time, the true remedies of the several patients suffering from such chronic affections.

§ 104

When the totality of the symptoms that specially mark and distinguish the case of disease or, in other words, when the picture of the disease, whatever be its kind, is once accurately sketched, [98] the most difficult part of the task is accomplished. The physician has then the picture of the disease, especially if it be a chronic one, always before him to guide him in his treatment; he can investigate it in all its parts and can pick out the characteristic symptoms, in order to oppose to these, that is to say, to the whole malady itself, a very similar artificial morbific force, in the shape of a homoeopathically chosen medicinal substance, selected from the lists of symptoms of all the medicines whose pure effects have been ascertained. And when, during the treatment, he wishes to ascertain what has been the effect of the medicine, and what change has taken place in the patient's state, at this fresh examination of the patient he only needs to strike out of the list of the symptoms noted down at the first visit those that have become ameliorated, to mark what still remain, and add any new symptoms that may have supervened.

§ 105

The second point of the business of a true physician related to acquiring a knowledge of the instruments intended for the cure of the natural diseases, investigating the pathogenetic power of the medicines, in order, when called on to cure, to be able to select from among them one, from the list of whose symptoms an artificial disease may be constructed, as similar as possible to the totality of the principal symptoms of the natural disease sought to be cured.

§ 106

The whole pathogenetic effect of the several medicines must be known; that is to say, all the morbid symptoms and alterations in the health that each of them is specially capable of developing in the healthy individual must first have been observed as far as possible, before we can hope to be able to find among them, and to select, suitable homoeopathic remedies for most of the natural disease.

§ 107

If, in order to ascertain this, medicines be given to sick persons only, even though they be administered singly and alone, then little or nothing precise is seen of their true effects, as those peculiar alterations of the health to be expected from the medicine are mixed up with the symptoms of the disease and can seldom be distinctly observed.

§ 108

There is, therefore, no other possible way in which the peculiar effects of medicines on the health of individuals can be accurately ascertained – there is no sure, no more natural way of accomplishing this object, than to administer the several medicines experimentally, in moderate doses, to healthy persons, in order to ascertain what changes, symptoms and signs of their influence each individually produces on the health of the body and of the mind; that is to say, what disease elements they are able and tend to produce, [99] since, as has been demonstrated (§§ 24-27), all the curative power of medicines lies in this power they possess of changing the state of man's health, and is revealed by observation of the latter.

§ 109

I was the first that opened up this path, which I have pursued with a perseverance that could only arise and be kept up by a perfect conviction of the great truth, fraught with such blessings to humanity, that it is only by the homoeopathic employment of medicines [100] that the certain cure of human maladies is possible. [101]

§ 110

I saw, moreover, that the morbid lesions which previous authors had observed to result from medicinal substances when taken into the stomach of healthy persons, either in large doses given by mistake or in order to produce death in themselves or others, or under other circumstances, accorded very much with my own observations when experimenting with the same substances on myself and other healthy individuals. These authors give details of what occurred as histories of poisoning and as proofs of the pernicious effects of these powerful substances, chiefly in order to warn others from their use; partly also for the sake of exalting their own skill, when, under the use of the remedies they employed to combat these dangerous accidents, health gradually returned; but partly also, when the persons so affected died under their treatment, in order to seek their own justification in the dangerous character of these substances, which they then termed poisons. None of these observers ever dreamed that the symptoms they recorded merely as proofs of the noxious and poisonous character of these substances were sure revelations of the power of these drugs to extinguish curatively similar symptoms occurring in natural disease, that these their pathogenetic phenomena were intimations of their homoeopathic curative action, and that the only possible way to ascertain their medicinal powers is to observe those changes of health medicines are capable of producing in the healthy organism; for the pure, peculiar powers of medicines available for the cure of disease are to be learned neither by any ingenious a priori speculations, nor by the smell, taste or appearance of the drugs, nor by their chemical analysis, nor yet by the employment of several of them at one time in a mixture (prescription) in diseases; it was never suspected that these histories of medicinal diseases would one day furnish the first rudiments of the true, pure materia medica, which from the earliest times until now has consisted solely of false conjectures and fictions of the imagination – that is to say, did not exist at all. [102]

§ 111

The agreement of my observations on the pure effects of medicines with these older ones – although they were recorded without reference to any therapeutic object, – and the very concordance of these accounts with others of the same kind by different authors must easily convince us that medicinal substances act in the morbid changes they produce in the healthy human body according to fixed, eternal laws of nature, and by virtue of these are enabled to produce certain, reliable disease symptoms each according to its own peculiar character.

§ 112

In those older prescriptions of the often dangerous effects of medicines ingested in excessively large doses we notice certain states that were produced, not at the commencement, but towards the termination of these sad events, and which were of an exactly opposite nature to those that first appeared. These symptoms, the very reverse of the primary action (§ 63) or proper action of the medicines on the vital force are the reaction of the vital force of the organism, its secondary action (§§ 62-67), of which, however, there is seldom or hardly ever the least trace from experiments with moderate doses on healthy bodies, and from small doses none whatever. In the homoeopathic curative operation the living organism reacts from these only so much as is requisite to raise the health again to the normal healthy state (§ 67).

§ 113
The only exceptions to this are the narcotic medicines. As they, in their primary action, take away sometimes the sensibility and sensation, sometimes the irritability, it frequently happens that in their secondary action, even from moderate experimental doses on healthy bodies, an increased sensibility (and a greater irritability) is observable.

§ 114
With the exception of these narcotic substances, in experiments with moderate doses of medicine on healthy bodies, we observe only their primary action, i.e., those symptoms wherewith the medicine deranges the health of the human being and develops in him a morbid state of longer or shorter duration.

§ 115
Among these symptoms, there occur in the case of some medicines not a few which are partially, or under certain conditions, directly opposite to other symptoms that have previously or subsequently appeared, but which are not therefore to be regarded as actual secondary action or the mere reaction of the vital force, but which only represent the alternating state of the various paroxysms of the primary action; they are termed alternating actions.

§ 116
Some symptoms are produced by the medicines more frequently – that is to say, in many individuals, others more rarely or in few persons, some only in very few healthy bodies.

§ 117
To the latter category belong the so-called idiosyncrasies, by which are meant peculiar corporeal constitutions which, although otherwise healthy, possess a disposition to be brought into a more or less morbid state by certain things which seem to produce no impression and no change in many other individuals. [103] But this inability to make an impression on every one is only apparent. For as two things are required for the production of these as well as all other morbid alterations in the health of man – to wit., the inherent power of the influencing substance, and the capability of the vital force that animates the organism to be influenced by it – the obvious derangements of health in the so-called idiosyncrasies cannot be laid to the account of these peculiar constitutions alone, but they must also be ascribed to these things that produce them, in which must lie the power of making the same impressions on all human bodies, yet in such a manner that but a small number of healthy constitutions have a tendency to allow themselves to be brought into such an obvious morbid condition by them. That these agents do actually make this impression on every healthy body is shown by this, that when employed as remedies they render effectual homoeopathic service [104] to all sick persons for morbid symptoms similar to those they seem to be only capable of producing in so-called idiosyncratic individuals.

§ 118
Every medicine exhibits peculiar actions on the human frame, which are not produced in exactly the same manner by any other medicinal substance of a different kind. [105]

§ 119

As certainly as every species of plant differs in its external form, mode of life and growth, in its taste and smell from every other species and genus of plant, as certainly as every mineral and salt differs from all others, in its external as well as its internal physical and chemical properties (which alone should have sufficed to prevent any confounding of one with another), so certainly do they all differ and diverge among themselves in their pathogenetic – consequently also in their therapeutic – effects. [106] Each of these substances produces alterations in the health of human beings in a peculiar, different, yet determinate manner, so as to preclude the possibility of confounding one with another. [107]

§ 120

Therefore medicines, on which depend man's life and death, disease and health, must be thoroughly and most carefully distinguished from one another, and for this purpose tested by careful, pure experiments on the healthy body for the purpose of ascertaining their powers and real effects, in order to obtain an accurate knowledge of them, and to enable us to avoid any mistake in their employment in diseases, for it is only by correct selection of them that the greatest of all earthly blessings, the health of the body and of the mind, can be rapidly and permanently restored.

§ 121

In proving medicines to ascertain their effects on the healthy body, it must be borne in mind that the strong, heroic substances, as they are termed, are liable even in small doses to produce changes in the health even of robust persons. Those of milder power must be given for these experiments in more considerable quantities; in order to observe the action of the very weakest, however, the subjects of experiment should be persons free from disease, and who are delicate, irritable and sensitive.

§ 122

In these experiments – on which depends the exactitude of the whole medical art, and the weal of all future generations of mankind – no other medicines should be employed except such as are perfectly well known, and of whose purity, genuineness and energy we are thoroughly assured.

§ 123

Each of these medicines must be taken in a perfectly simple, unadulterated form; the indigenous plants in the form of freshly expressed juice, mixed with a little alcohol to prevent it spoiling; exotic vegetable substances, however, in the form of powder, or tincture prepared with alcohol when they were in the fresh state and afterwards mingled with a certain proportion of water; salts and gums, however, should be dissolved in water just before being taken. If the plant can only be procured in its dry state, and if its powers are naturally weak, in that case there may be used for the experiment an infusion of it, made by cutting the herb into small pieces and pouring boiling water on it, so as to extract its medicinal parts; immediately after its preparation it must be swallowed while still warm, as all expressed vegetable juices and all aqueous infusions of herbs, without the addition of spirit, pass rapidly into fermentation and decomposition, whereby all their medicinal properties are lost.

§ 124

For these experiments every medicinal substance must be employed quite alone and perfectly pure, without the admixture of any foreign substance, and without taking anything else of a medicinal nature the same day, nor yet on the subsequent days, nor during all the time we wish to observe the effects of the medicine.

§ 125

During all the time the experiment lasts the diet must be strictly regulated; it should be as much as possible destitute of spices, of a purely nutritious and simple character, green vegetables, [108] roots and all salads and herb soups (which, even when most carefully prepared, possess some disturbing medicinal qualities) should be avoided. The drinks are to be those usually partaken of, as little stimulating as possible. [109]

§ 126 Fifth Edition

The person who is proving the medicine must during the whole time of the experiment avoid all over-exertion of mind and body, all sorts of dissipation and disturbing passions; he should have no urgent business to distract his attention; he must devote himself to careful self-observation and not be disturbed while so engaged; his body must be in what is for him a good state of health, and he must possess a sufficient amount of intelligence to be able to express and describe his sensations in accurate terms.

§ 126 Sixth Edition

The person who is proving the medicine must be pre-eminently trustworthy and conscientious and during the whole time of the experiment avoid all over-exertion of mind and body, all sorts of dissipation and disturbing passions; he should have no urgent business to distract his attention; he must devote himself to careful self-observation and not be disturbed while so engaged; his body must be in what is for him a good state of health, and he must possess a sufficient amount of intelligence to be able to express and describe his sensations in accurate terms.

§ 127

The medicines must be tested on both males and females, in order also to reveal the alterations of the health they produce in the sexual sphere.

§ 128 Fifth Edition

The most recent observations have shown that medicinal substances, when taken in their crude state by the experimenter for the purpose of testing their peculiar effects, do not exhibit nearly the full amount of the powers that lie hidden in them which they do when they are taken for the same object in high dilutions potentized by proper trituration and succussion, by which simple operations the powers which in their crude state lay hidden, and, as it were, dormant, are developed and roused into activity to an incredible extent. In this manner we now find it best to investigate the medicinal powers even of such substances as are deemed weak, and the plan we adopt is to give to the experimenter, on an empty stomach, daily from four to six very small globules of the thirtieth potentized dilution of such a substance, moistened with a little water, and let him continue this for several days.

§ 128 Sixth Edition

The most recent observations have shown that medicinal substances, when taken in their crude state by the experimenter for the purpose of testing their peculiar effects, do not exhibit nearly the full amount of the powers that lie hidden in them which they do when they are taken for the same object in high dilutions potentized by proper trituration and succussion, by which simple operations the powers which in their crude state lay hidden, and, as it were, dormant, are developed and roused into activity to an incredible extent. In this manner we now find it best to investigate the medicinal powers even of such substances as are deemed weak, and the plan we adopt is to give to the experimenter, on an empty stomach, daily from four to six very small globules of the thirtieth potency of such a substance, moistened with a little water or dissolved in more or less water and thoroughly mixed, and let him continue this for several days.

§ 129

If the effects that result from such a dose are but slight, a few more globules may be taken daily, until they become more distinct and stronger and the alterations of the health more conspicuous; for all persons are not effected by a medicine in an equally great degree; on the contrary, there is a vast variety in this respect, so that sometimes an apparently weak individual may by scarcely at all affected by moderate doses of a medicine known to be of a powerful character, while he is strongly enough acted on by others of a much weaker kind. And, on the other hand, there are very robust persons who experience very considerable morbid symptoms from an apparently mild medicine, and only slighter symptoms from stronger drugs. Now, as this cannot be known beforehand, it is advisable to commence in every instance with a small dose of the drug and, where suitable and requisite, to increase the dose more and more from day to day.

§ 130

If, at the very commencement, the first dose administered shall have been sufficiently strong, this advantage is gained, that the experimenter learns the order of succession of the symptoms and can note down accurately the period at which each occurs, which is very useful in leading to a knowledge of the genius of the medicine, for then the order of the primary actions, as also that of the alternating actions, is observed in the most unambiguous manner. A very moderate dose, even, often suffices for the experiment, provided only the experimenter is endowed with sufficiently delicate sensitiveness, and is very attentive to his sensations. The duration of the action of a drug can only be ascertained by a comparison of several experiments.

§ 131

If, however, in order to ascertain anything at all, the same medicine must be given to the same person to test for several successive days in ever increasing doses, we thereby learn, no doubt, the various morbid states this medicine is capable of producing in a general manner, but we do not ascertain their order of succession; and the subsequent dose often removes, curatively, some one or other of the symptoms caused by the previous dose, or develops in its stead an opposite state; such symptoms should be enclosed in brackets, to mark their ambiguity, until subsequent purer experiments show whether they are the reaction of the organism and secondary action or an alternating action of this medicine.

§ 132

But when the object is, without reference to the sequential order of the phenomena and the duration of the action of the drug, only to ascertain the symptoms themselves, especially those of a weak medicinal substance, in that case the preferable course to pursue is to give it for several successive days, increasing the dose every day. In this manner the action of an unknown medicine, even of the mildest nature, will be revealed, especially if tested on sensitive persons.

§ 133

On experiencing any particular sensation from the medicine, it is useful, indeed necessary, in order to determine the exact character of the symptom, to assume various positions while it lasts, and to observe whether, by moving the part affected, by walking in the room or the open air, by standing, sitting or lying the symptom is increased, diminished or removed, and whether it returns on again assuming the position in which it was first observed, – whether it is altered by eating or drinking, or by any other condition, or by speaking, coughing, sneezing or any other action of the body, and at the same time to note at what time of the day or night it usually occurs in the most marked manner, whereby what is peculiar to and characteristic of each symptom will become apparent.

§ 134

All external influences, and more especially medicines, possess the property of producing in the health of the living organism a particular kind of alteration peculiar to themselves; but all the symptoms peculiar to a medicine do not appear in one person, nor all at once, nor in the same experiment, but some occur in one person chiefly at one time, others again during a second or third trail; in another person some other symptoms appear, but in such a manner that probably some of the phenomena are observed in the fourth, eighth or tenth person which had already appeared in the second, sixth or ninth person, and so forth; moreover, they may not recur at the same hour.

§ 135

The whole of the elements of disease a medicine is capable of producing can only be brought to anything like completeness by numerous observations on suitable persons of both sexes and of various constitutions. We can only be assured that a medicine has been thoroughly proved in regard to the morbid states it can produce – that is to say, in regard to its pure powers of altering the health of man – when subsequent experimenters can notice little of a novel character from its action, and almost always only the same symptoms as had been already observed by others.

§ 136

Although, as has been said, a medicine, on being proved on healthy subjects, cannot develop in one person all the alterations of health it is capable of causing, but can only do this when given to many different individuals, varying in their corporeal and mental constitution, yet the tendency to excite all these symptoms in every human being exists in it (§ 117), according to an eternal and immutable law of nature, by virtue of which all its effects, even those that are but rarely developed in the healthy person, are brought into operation in the case of every individual if administered to him when he is in a morbid state presenting similar symptoms; it then, even in the smallest dose, being homoeopathically selected, silently produces in the patient an artificial state closely resembling the natural disease, which rapidly and permanently (homoeopathically) frees and cures him of his original malady.

§ 137

The more moderate, within certain limits, the doses of the medicine used for such experiments are – provided we endeavor to facilitate the observation by the selection of a person who is a lover of truth, temperate in all respects, of delicate feelings, and who can direct the most minute attention to his sensation – so much the more distinctly are the primary effects developed, and only these, which are most worth knowing, occur without any admixture of secondary effects or reactions of the vital force. When, however, excessively large doses are used there occur at the same time not only a number of secondary effects among the symptoms, but the primary effects developed, and only these, which are most worth knowing, occur without any admixture of secondary effects or reactions of the vital force. When, however, excessively large doses are used there occur at the same time not only a number of secondary effects among the symptoms, but the primary effects also come on in such hurried confusion and with such impetuosity that nothing can be accurately observed; let alone the danger attending them, which no one who has any regard for his fellow-creatures, and who looks on the meanest of mankind as his brother, will deem an indifferent manner.

§ 138

All the sufferings, accidents and changes of the health of the experimenter during the action of a medicine (provided the above condition [§§ 124-127] essential to a good and pure experiment are complied with) are solely derived from this medicine, and must be regarded and registered as belonging peculiarly to this medicine, as symptoms of this medicine, even though the experimenter had observed, a considerable time previously, the spontaneous occurrence of similar phenomena in himself. The reappearance of these during the trial of the medicine only shows that this individual is, by virtue of his peculiar constitution, particularly disposed to have such symptoms excited in him. In this case they are the effect of the medicine; the symptoms do not arise spontaneously while the medicine that has been taken is exercising an influence over the health of the whole system, but are produced by the medicine.

§ 139

When the physician does not make the trial of the medicine on himself, but gives it to another person, the latter must note down distinctly the sensations, sufferings, accidents and changes of health he experiences at the time of their occurrence, mentioning the time after the ingestion of the drug when each symptom arose and, if it lasts long, the period of its duration. The physician looks over the report in the presence of the experimenter immediately after the experiment is concluded, or if the trial lasts several days he does this every day, in order, while everything is still fresh in his memory, to question him about the exact nature of every one of these circumstances, and to write down the more precise details so elicited, or to make such alterations as the experimenter may suggest. [110]

§ 140

If the person cannot write, the physician must be informed by him every day of what has occurred to him, and how it took place. What is noted down as authentic information on this point, however, must be chiefly the voluntary narration of the person who makes the experiment, nothing conjectural and as little as possible derived from answers to leading questions should be admitted; everything must be ascertained with the same caution as I have counselled above (§§ 84-99) for the investigation of the phenomena and for tracing the picture of natural diseases.

§ 141
But the best provings of the pure effects of simple medicines in altering the human health, and of the artificial diseases and symptoms they are capable of developing in the healthy individual, are those which the healthy, unprejudiced and sensitive physician institutes on himself with all the caution and care here enjoined. He knows with the greatest certainty the things he has experienced in his own person. [111]

§ 142
But how some symptoms1 of the simple medicine employed for a curative purpose can be distinguished amongst the symptoms of the original malady, even in diseases, especially in those of a chronic character that usually remain unaltered, is a subject appertaining to the higher art of judgement, and must be left exclusively to masters in observation.

§ 143
If we have thus tested on the healthy individual a considerable number of simple medicines and carefully and faithfully registered all the disease elements and symptoms they are capable of developing as artificial disease-producers, then only have we a true materia medica – a collection of real, pure, reliable [113] modes of action of simple medicinal substances, a volume of the book of nature, wherein is recorded a considerable array of the peculiar changes of the health and symptoms ascertained to belong to each of the powerful medicines, as they were revealed to the attention of the observer, in which the likeness of the (homoeopathic) disease elements of many natural diseases to be hereafter cured by them are present, which, in a word, contain artificial morbid states, that furnish for the similar natural morbid states the only true, homoeopathic, that is to say, specific, therapeutic instruments for effecting their certain and permanent cure.

§ 144
From such a materia medica everything that is conjectural, all that is mere assertion or imaginary should be strictly excluded; everything should be the pure language of nature carefully and honestly interrogated.

§ 145 Fifth Edition
Of a truth, it is only by a very considerable store of medicines accurately known in respect of these their pure modes of action in altering the health of man, that we can be placed in a position to discover a homoeopathic remedy, a suitable artificial (curative) morbific analogue for each of the infinitely numerous morbid states in nature, for every malady in the world. [114] In the meantime, even now – thanks to the truthful character of the symptoms, and to the abundance of disease elements which every one of the powerful medicinal substances has already shown in its action on the healthy body – but few disease remain, for which a tolerably suitable homoeopathic remedy may not be met with among those now proved as to their pure action, [115] which, without much disturbance, restores health in a gentle, sure and permanent manner - infinitely more surely and safe-

ly than can be effected by all the general and special therapeutics of the old allopathic medical art with its unknown composite remedies, which do but alter and aggravate but cannot cure chronic diseases, and rather retard than promote recovery from acute diseases.

§ 145 Sixth Edition

Of a truth, it is only by a very considerable store of medicines accurately known in respect of these their pure modes of action in altering the health of man, that we can be placed in a position to discover a homoeopathic remedy, a suitable artificial (curative) morbific analogue for each of the infinitely numerous morbid states in nature, for every malady in the world. [116] In the meantime, even now – thanks to the truthful character of the symptoms, and to the abundance of disease elements which every one of the powerful medicinal substances has already shown in its action on the healthy body – but few disease remain, for which a tolerably suitable homoeopathic remedy may not be met with among those now proved as to their pure action, [115] which, without much disturbance, restores health in a gentle, sure and permanent manner - infinitely more surely and safely than can be effected by all the general and special therapeutics of the old allopathic medical art with its unknown composite remedies, which do but alter and aggravate but cannot cure chronic diseases, and rather retard than promote recovery from acute diseases and frequently endanger life.

§ 146

The third point of the business of a true physician relates to the judicious employment of the artificial morbific agents (medicines) that have been proved on healthy individuals to ascertain their pure action in order to effect the homoeopathic cure of natural diseases.

§ 147

Whichever of these medicines that have been investigated as to their power of altering man's health we find to contain in the symptoms observed from its use the greatest similarity to the totality of the symptoms of a given natural disease, this medicine will and must be the most suitable, the most certain homoeopathic remedy for the disease; in it is found the specific remedy of this case of disease.

§ 148 Fifth Edition

A medicine selected in this manner, which has the power and the tendency to produce symptoms the most similar possible to the disease to be cured, consequently a similar artificial disease, given in a suitable dose, affects, in its dynamic action on the morbidly deranged vital force of the individual, those very parts and points in the organism now suffering from the natural disease, and produces in them its own artificial disease, which, on account of its great similarity and preponderating strength, occupies precisely the seat hitherto occupied by the natural morbid derangement, so that the instinctive, automatic vital force is from that time forward no longer affected by the natural disease but solely by the stronger, similar medicinal disease; which in its turn, on account of the small dose of the remedy, being, like every moderate medicinal disease, overcome by the increased energy of the vital force, soon spontaneously disappears, leaving the body free from all disease, that is to say, healthy and permanently cured.

§ 148 Sixth Edition

The natural disease is never to be considered as a noxious material situated somewhere within the interior or exterior of man (§ 11-13) but as one produced by an inimical spirit-like (conceptual) agency which, like a kind of infection (note to § 11) disturbs in its instinctive existence of the spirit-like (conceptual) principle of life within the organism torturing it as an evil spirit and compelling it to produce certain ailments and disorders in the regular course of its life. These are known as symptoms (disease). If, now, the influence of this inimical agency that not only caused but strives to continue this disorder, be taken away as is done when the physician administers an artificial potency, capable of altering the life principle in the most similar manner (a homoeopathic medicine) which exceeds in energy even in the smallest dose the similar natural disease (§§ 33, 279), then the influence of the original noxious morbid agent on the life principle is lost during the action of this stronger similar artificial disease. Thence the evil no longer exists for the life principle – it is destroyed. If, as has been said, the selected homoeopathic remedy is administered properly, then the acute natural disease which is to be overruled if recently developed, will disappear imperceptibly in a few hours.

An older, more chronic disease will yield somewhat later together with all traces of discomfort, by the use of several doses of the same more highly potentized remedy or after careful selection [117] of one or another more similar homoeopathic medicine. Health, recovery, follow in imperceptible, often rapid transitions. The life principle is freed again and capable of resuming the life of the organism in health as before and strength returns.

§ 149 Fifth Edition

When the suitable homoeopathic remedy has been thus selected and rightly employed, the acute disease we wish to cure, even though it be of a grave character and attended by many sufferings subsides insensibly, in a few hours if it be of recent date, in a few days if it be of a somewhat longer standing, along with all traces of indisposition, and nothing or almost nothing more of the artificial medicinal disease is perceived; there occurs, by rapid, imperceptible transitions, noting but restored health, recovery. Disease of long standing (and especially such as are of a complicated character) require for their cure a proportionately longer time. More especially do the chronic medicinal dyscrasia so often produced by allopathic bungling, along with the natural disease left uncured by it, require a much longer time for their recovery; often, indeed, are they incurable, in consequence of the shameful robbery of the patient's strength and juices, the principal feat performed by allopathy in its so-called methods of treatment.

§ 149 Sixth Edition

Diseases of long standing (and especially such as are of a complicated character) require for their cure a proportionately longer time. More especially do the chronic medicinal dyscrasia so often produced by allopathic bungling along with the natural disease left uncured by it, require a much longer time for their recovery; often, indeed, are they incurable, in consequence of the shameful robbery of the patient's strength and juices (venesections, purgatives, etc.), on account of long continued use of large doses of violently acting remedies given on the basis of empty, false theories for alleged usefulness in cases of disease appearing similar, also in prescribing unsuitable mineral baths, etc., the principal feat performed by allopathy in its so-called methods of treatment.

§ 150
If a patient complain of one or more trivial symptoms, that have been only observed a short time previously, the physician should not regard this as a fully developed disease but requires serious medical aid. A slight alteration in the diet and regimen will usually suffice to dispel such an indisposition.

§ 151
But if the patient complain of a few violent sufferings, the physician will usually find, on investigation, several other symptoms besides, although of a slighter character, which furnish a complete picture of the disease.

§ 152
The worse of the acute disease is, of so much the more numerous and striking symptoms is it generally composed, but with so much the more certainly may a suitable remedy for it be found, if there be a sufficient number of medicines known, with respect to their positive action, to choose from. Among the lists of symptoms of many medicines it will not be difficult to find one from whose separate disease elements an antitype of curative artificial disease, very like the totality of the symptoms of the natural disease, may be constructed, and such a medicine is the desired remedy.

§ 153 Fifth Edition
In this search for a homoeopathic specific remedy, that is to say, in this comparison of the collective symptoms of the natural disease with the list of symptoms of known medicines, in order to find among these an artificial morbific agent corresponding by similarity to the disease to be cured, the more striking, singular, uncommon and peculiar (characteristic) signs and symptoms [118] of the case of disease are chiefly and most solely to be kept in view; for it is more particularly these that very similar ones in the list of symptoms of the selected medicine must correspond to, in order to constitute it the most suitable for effecting the cure. The more general and undefined symptoms: loss of appetite, headache, debility, restless sleep, discomfort, and so forth, demand but little attention when of that vague and indefinite character, if they cannot be more accurately described, as symptoms of such a general nature are observed in almost every disease and from almost every drug.

§ 153 Sixth Edition
In this search for a homoeopathic specific remedy, that is to say, in this comparison of the collective symptoms of the natural disease with the list of symptoms of known medicines, in order to find among these an artificial morbific agent corresponding by similarity to the disease to be cured, the more striking, singular, uncommon and peculiar (characteristic) signs and symptoms [119] of the case of disease are chiefly and most solely to be kept in view; for it is more particularly these that very similar ones in the list of symptoms of the selected medicine must correspond to, in order to constitute it the most suitable for effecting the cure. The more general and undefined symptoms: loss of appetite, headache, debility, restless sleep, discomfort, and so forth, demand but little attention when of that vague and indefinite character, if they cannot be more accurately de-

scribed, as symptoms of such a general nature are observed in almost every disease and from almost every drug.

§ 154
If the antitype constructed from the list of symptoms of the most suitable medicine contain those peculiar, uncommon, singular and distinguishing (characteristic) symptoms, which are to be met with in the disease to be cured in the greatest number and in the greatest similarity, this medicine is the most appropriate homoeopathic specific remedy for this morbid state; the disease, if it be not one of very long standing, will generally be removed and extinguished by the first dose of it, without any considerable disturbance.

§ 155 Fifth Edition
I say without any considerable disturbance. For in the employment of this most appropriate homoeopathic remedy it is only the symptoms of the medicine that correspond to the symptoms of the disease that are called into play, the former occupying the place of the latter (weaker) in the organism, and thereby annihilating them by overpowering them; but the other symptoms of the homoeopathic medicine, which are often very numerous, being in no way applicable to the case of disease in question, are not called into play at all. The patient, growing hourly better, feels almost nothing of them at all, because the excessively minute dose requisite for homoeopathic use is much too weak to produce the other symptoms of the medicine that are not homoeopathic to the case, in those parts of the body that are free from disease, and consequently can allow only the homoeopathic symptoms to act on the parts of the organism that are already most irritated and excited by the similar symptoms of the disease, thus changing the morbid affection of the vital force into a similar but stronger medicinal disease, whereby the original malady is extinguished.

§ 155 Sixth Edition
I say without any considerable disturbance. For in the employment of this most appropriate homoeopathic remedy it is only the symptoms of the medicine that correspond to the symptoms of the disease that are called into play, the former occupying the place of the latter (weaker) in the organism, i.e., in the sensation of the life principle, and thereby annihilating them by overpowering them; but the other symptoms of the homoeopathic medicine, which are often very numerous, being in no way applicable to the case of disease in question, are not called into play at all. The patient, growing hourly better, feels almost nothing of them at all, because the excessively minute dose requisite for homoeopathic use is much too weak to produce the other symptoms of the medicine that are not homoeopathic to the case, in those parts of the body that are free from disease, and consequently can allow only the homoeopathic symptoms to act on the parts of the organism that are already most irritated and excited by the similar symptoms of the disease, in order that the sick life principle may react only to a similar but stronger medicinal disease, whereby the original malady is extinguished.

§ 156
There is, however, almost no homoeopathic medicine, be it ever so suitably chosen, that, especially if it should be given in an insufficiently minute dose, will not produce, in very irritable and sensitive patients, at least one trifling, unusual disturbance, some slight new symptom while its action lasts; for it is next to impos-

sible that medicine and disease should cover one another symptomatically as exactly as two triangles with equal sides and equal angles. But this (in ordinary circumstances) unimportant difference will be easily done away with by the potential activity (energy) of the living organism, and is not perceptible by patients not excessively delicate; the restoration goes forward, notwithstanding, to the goal of perfect recovery, if it be not prevented by the action of heterogeneous medicinal influences upon the patient, by errors of regimen or by excitement of the passions.

§ 157 Fifth Edition

But though it is certain that a homoeopathically selected remedy does, by reason of its appropriateness and the minuteness of the dose, gently remove and annihilate the acute disease analogous to it, without manifesting its other unhomoeopathic symptoms, that is to say, without the production of new, serious disturbances, yet it usually, immediately after ingestion – for the first hour, or for a few hours – causes a kind of slight aggravation (where the dose has been somewhat too large, however, for a considerable number of hours), which has so much resemblance to the original disease that it seems to the patient to be an aggravation of his own disease. But it is, in reality, nothing more than an extremely similar medicinal disease, somewhat exceeding in strength the original affection.

§ 157 Sixth Edition

But though it is certain that a homoeopathically selected remedy does, by reason of its appropriateness and the minuteness of the dose, gently remove and annihilate the acute disease analogous to it, without manifesting its other unhomoeopathic symptoms, that is to say, without the production of new, serious disturbances, yet it usually, immediately after ingestion – for the first hour, or for a few hours – causes a kind of slight aggravation when the dose has not been sufficiently small and (where the dose has been somewhat too large, however, for a considerable number of hours), which has so much resemblance to the original disease that it seems to the patient to be an aggravation of his own disease. But it is, in reality, nothing more than an extremely similar medicinal disease, somewhat exceeding in strength the original affection.

§ 158

This slight homoeopathic aggravation during the first hours – a very good prognostic that the acute disease will most probably yield to the first dose – is quite as it ought to be, as the medicinal disease must naturally be somewhat stronger than the malady to be cured if it is to overpower and extinguish the latter, just as a natural disease can remove and annihilate another one similar to it only when it is stronger than the latter (§§ 43 – 48).

§ 159 Fifth Edition

The smaller the dose of the homoeopathic remedy is, so much the slighter and shorter is the apparent increase of the disease during the first hours.

§ 159 Sixth Edition

The smaller the dose of the homoeopathic remedy is in the treatment of acute diseases so much the slighter and shorter is the apparent increase of the disease during the first hours.

§ 160

But as the dose of a homoeopathic remedy can scarcely ever be made so small that it shall not be able to relieve, overpower, indeed completely cure and annihilate the uncomplicated natural disease of not long standing that is analogous to it (§ 249, note), we can understand why a does of an appropriate homoeopathic medicine, not the very smallest possible, does always, during the first hour after its ingestion, produce a perceptible homoeopathic aggravation of this kind. [120]

§ 161 Sixth Edition

When I here limit the so-called homoeopathic aggravation, or rather the primary action of the homoeopathic medicine that seems to increase somewhat the symptoms of the original disease, to the first or few hours, this is certainly true with respect to diseases of a more acute character and of recent origin, but where medicines of long action have to combat a malady of, considerable or of very long standing, where no such apparent increase of the original disease ought to appear during treatment and it does not so appear if the accurately chosen medicine was given in proper small, gradually higher doses, each somewhat modified with renewed dynamization (§ 247). Such increase of the original symptoms of a chronic disease can appear only at the end of treatment when the cure is almost or quite finished.

§ 162

Sometimes happens, owing to the moderate number of medicines yet known with respect to their true, pure action , that but a portion of the symptoms of the disease under treatment are to be met with in the list of symptoms of the most appropriate medicine, consequently this imperfect medicinal morbific agent must be employed for lack of a more perfect one.

§ 163

In this case we cannot indeed expect from this medicine a complete, untroubled cure; for during its use some symptoms appear which were not previously observable in the disease, accessory symptoms of the not perfectly appropriate remedy. This does by no means prevent a considerable part of the disease (the symptoms of the disease that resemble those of the medicine) from being eradicated by this medicine, thereby establishing a fair commencement of the cure, but still this does not take place without those accessory symptoms, which are, however, always moderate when the dose of the medicine is sufficiently minute.

§ 164

The small number of homoeopathic symptoms present in the best selected medicine is no obstacle to the cure in cases where these few medicinal symptoms are chiefly of an uncommon kind and such as are peculiarly distinctive (characteristic) of the disease; the cure takes place under such circumstances without any particular disturbance.

§ 165

If, however, among the symptoms of the remedy selected, there be none that accurately resemble the distinctive (characteristic), peculiar, uncommon symptoms of the case of disease, and if the remedy correspond to the disease only in the general, vaguely described, indefinite states (nausea, debility, headache, and so forth), and if there be among the known medicines none more homoeopathically appropriate, in that case the physician cannot promise himself any immediate favorable result from the employment of this unhomoeopathic medicine.

§ 166

Such a case is, however, very rare, owing to the increased number of medicines whose pure effects are now known, and the bad effects resulting from it, when they do occur, are diminished whenever a subsequent medicine, of more accurate resemblance, can be selected.

§ 167

Thus if there occur, during the use of this imperfectly homoeopathic remedy first employed, accessory symptoms of some moment, then, in the case of acute diseases, we do not allow this first dose to exhaust its action, nor leave the patient to the full duration of the action of the remedy, but we investigate afresh the morbid state in its now altered condition, and add the remainder of the original symptoms to those newly developed in tracing a new picture of the disease.

§ 168

We shall then be able much more readily to discover, among the known medicines, an analogue to the morbid state before us, a single dose of which, if it do not entirely destroy the disease, will advance it considerably on the way to be cured. And thus we go on, if even this medicine be not quite sufficient to effect the restoration of health, examining again and again the morbid state that still remains, and selecting a homoeopathic medicine as suitable as possible for it, until our object, namely, putting the patient in the possession of perfect health, is accomplished.

§ 169 Fifth Edition

If, on the first examination of a disease and the first selection of a medicine, we should find that the totality of the symptoms of the disease would not be effectually covered by the disease elements of a single medicine – owing to the insufficient number of known medicines, – but that two medicines contend for the preference in point of appropriateness, one of which is more homoeopathically suitable for one part, the other for another part of the symptoms of the disease, it is not advisable, after the employment of the more suitable of the two medicines, to administer the other without fresh examination, for the medicine that seemed to be the next best would not, under the change of circumstances that has in the meantime taken place, be suitable for the rest of the symptoms that then remain; in which case, consequently, a more appropriate homoeopathic remedy must be selected in place of the second medicine for the set of symptoms as they appear on a new inspection.

§ 169 Sixth Edition

If, on the first examination of a disease and the first selection of a medicine, we should find that the totality of the symptoms of the disease would not be effectually covered by the disease elements of a single medicine – owing to the insufficient number of known medicines, – but that two medicines contend for the preference in point of appropriateness, one of which is more homoeopathically suitable for one part, the other for another part of the symptoms of the disease, it is not advisable, after the employment of the more suitable of the two medicines, to administer the other without fresh examination, and much less to give both together (§ 272, note) for the medicine that seemed to be the next best would not, under the change of circumstances that has in the meantime taken place, be suitable for the rest of the symptoms that then remain; in which case, consequently, a more appropriate homoeopathic remedy must be selected in place of the second medicine for the set of symptoms as they appear on a new inspection.

§ 170
Hence in this as in every case where a change of the morbid state has occurred, the remaining set of symptoms now present must be inquired into, and (without paying any attention to the medicine which at first appeared to be the next in point of suitableness) another homoeopathic medicine, as appropriate as possible to the new state now before us, must be selected. If it should so happen, as is not often the case, that the medicine which at first appeared to be the next best seems still to be well adapted for the morbid state that remains, so much the more will it merit our confidence, and deserve to be employed in preference to another.

§ 171 Fifth Edition
In non-venereal chronic disease, those, therefore, that arise from psora, we often require, in order to effect a cure, to give several antipsoric remedies in succession, every successive one being homoeopathically chosen in consonance with the group of symptoms remaining after the expiry of the action of the previous remedy (which may have been employed in a single dose or in several successive doses).

§ 171 Sixth Edition
In non-venereal chronic disease, those, therefore, that arise from psora, we often require, in order to effect a cure, to give several antipsoric remedies in succession, every successive one being homoeopathically chosen in consonance with the group of symptoms remaining after completion of the action of the previous remedy.

§ 172
A similar difficulty in the way of the cure occurs from the symptoms of the disease being too few – a circumstances that deserves our careful attention, for by its removal almost all the difficulties that can lie in the way of this most perfect of all possible modes of treatment (except that its apparatus of known homoeopathic medicines is still incomplete) are removed.

§ 173
The only diseases that seem to have but few symptoms, and on that account to be less amenable to cure, are those which may be termed one-sided, because they display only one or two principal symptoms which obscure almost all the others. They belong chiefly to the class of chronic diseases.

§ 174
Their principal symptom may be either an internal complaint (e.g. a headache of many years' duration, a diarrhoea of long standing, an ancient cardialgia, etc.), or it may be an affection more of an external kind. Diseases of the latter character are generally distinguished by the name of local maladies.

§ 175
In one-sided diseases of the first kind it is often to be attributed to the medical observer's want of discernment that he does not fully discover the symptoms actually present which would enable him to complete the sketch of the portrait of the disease.

§ 176

There are, however, still a few diseases, which, after the most careful initial examination (§§ 84-98), present but one or two severe, violent symptoms, while all the others are but indistinctly perceptible.

§ 177
In order to meet most successfully such a case as this, which is of very rare occurrence, we are in the first place to select, guided by these few symptoms, the medicine which in our judgment is the most homoeopathically indicated.

§ 178
It will, no doubt, sometimes happen that this medicine, selected in strict observance of the homoeopathic law, furnishes the similar artificial disease suited for the annihilation of the malady present; and this is much more likely to happen when these few morbid symptoms are very striking, decided, uncommon and peculiarly distinctive (characteristic).

§ 179
More frequently, however, the medicine first chosen in such a case will be only partially, that is to say, not exactly suitable, as there was no considerable number of symptoms to guide to an accurate selection.

§ 180
In this case the medicine, which has been chosen as well as was possible, but which, for the reason above stated, is only imperfectly homoeopathic, will, in its action upon the disease that is only partially analogous to it – just as in the case mentioned above (§ 162, et seq.) where the limited number of homoeopathic remedies renders the selection imperfect – produce accessory symptoms, and several phenomena from its own array of symptoms are mixed up with the patient's state of health, which are, however, at the same time, symptoms of the disease itself, although they may have been hitherto never or very rarely perceived; some symptoms which the patient had never previously experienced appear, or others he had only felt indistinctly become more pronounced.

§ 181
Let is not be objected that the accessory phenomena and new symptoms of this disease that now appear should be laid to the account of the medicament just employed. They owe their origin to it [121] certainly, but they are always only symptoms of such a nature as this disease was itself capable of producing in this organism, and which were summoned forth and induced to make their appearance by the medicine given, owing to its power to cause similar symptoms. In a word, we have to regard the whole collection of symptoms now perceptible as belonging to the disease itself, as the actual existing condition, and to direct our further treatment accordingly.

§ 182
Thus the imperfect selection of the medicament, which was in this case almost inevitable owing to the too limited number of the symptoms present, serves to complete the display of the symptoms of the disease, and in this way facilitates the discovery of a second, more accurately suitable, homoeopathic medicine.

§ 183
Whenever, therefore, the dose of the first medicine ceases to have a beneficial effect (if the newly developed symptoms do not, by reason of their gravity, demand more speedy aid – which, however, from the minuteness of the dose of

homoeopathic medicine, and in very chronic diseases, is excessively rare), a new examination of the disease must be instituted, the status morbi as it now is must be noted down, and a second homoeopathic remedy selected in accordance with it, which shall exactly suit the present state, and one which shall be all the more appropriate can then be found, as the group of symptoms has become larger and more complete. [122]

§ 184 Fifth Edition

In like manner, after each new dose of medicine has exhausted its action, the state of the disease that still remains is to be noted anew with respect to its remaining symptoms, and another homoeopathic remedy sought for, as suitable as possible for the group of symptoms now observed, and so on until the recovery is complete.

§ 184 Sixth Edition

In like manner, after each new dose of medicine has exhausted its action, when it is no longer suitable and helpful, the state of the disease that still remains is to be noted anew with respect to its remaining symptoms, and another homoeopathic remedy sought for, as suitable as possible for the group of symptoms now observed, and so on until the recovery is complete.

§ 185

Among the one-sided disease an important place is occupied by the so-called local maladies, by which term is signified those changes and ailments that appear on the external parts of the body. Till now the idea prevalent in the schools was that these parts were alone morbidly affected, and that the rest of the body did not participate in the disease – a theoretical, absurd doctrine, which has led to the most disastrous medical treatment.

§ 186 Fifth Edition

Those so-called local maladies which have been produced a short time previously, solely by an external lesion, still appear at first sight to deserve the name of local disease. But then the lesion must be very trivial, and in that case it would be of no great moment. For in the case of injuries accruing to the body from without, if they be at all severe, the whole living organism sympathizes; there occur fever, etc. The treatment of such diseases is relegated to surgery; but this is right only in so far as the affected parts require mechanical aid, whereby the external obstacles to the cure, which can only be expected to take place by the agency of the vital force, may be removed by mechanical means, e.g., by the reduction of dislocations, by bandages to bring together the lips of wounds, by the extraction of foreign bodies that have penetrated into the living parts, by making an opening into a cavity of the body in order to remove an irritating substance or to procure the evacuation of effusions or collections of fluids, by bringing into apposition the broken extremities of a fractured bone and retaining them in exact contact by an appropriate bandage, etc. But when in such injuries the whole living organism requires, as it always does, active dynamic aid to put it in a position to accomplish the work of healing, e.g. when the violent fever resulting from extensive contusions, lacerated muscles, tendons and blood-vessels requires to be removed by medicine given internally, or when the external pain of scalded or burnt parts needs to be homoeopathically subdued, then the services of the dynamic physician and his helpful homoeopathy come into requisition.

§ 186 Sixth Edition

Those so-called local maladies which have been produced a short time previously, solely by an external lesion, still appear at first sight to deserve the name of local disease. But then the lesion must be very trivial, and in that case it would be of no great moment. For in the case of injuries accruing to the body from without, if they be at all severe, the whole living organism sympathizes; there occur fever, etc. The treatment of such diseases is relegated to surgery; but this is right only in so far as the affected parts require mechanical aid, whereby the external obstacles to the cure, which can only be expected to take place by the agency of the vital force, may be removed by mechanical means, e.g., by the reduction of dislocations, by needles and bandages to bring together the lips of wounds, by mechanical pressure to still the flow of blood from open arteries, by the extraction of foreign bodies that have penetrated into the living parts, by making an opening into a cavity of the body in order to remove an irritating substance or to procure the evacuation of effusions or collections of fluids, by bringing into apposition the broken extremities of a fractured bone and retaining them in exact contact by an appropriate bandage, etc. But when in such injuries the whole living organism requires, as it always does, active dynamic aid to put it in a position to accomplish the work of healing, e.g. when the violent fever resulting from extensive contusions, lacerated muscles, tendons and blood-vessels requires to be removed by medicine given internally, or when the external pain of scalded or burnt parts needs to be homoeopathically subdued, then the services of the dynamic physician and his helpful homoeopathy come into requisition.

§ 187

But those affections, alterations and ailments appearing on the external parts, that do not arise from any external injury or that have only some slight external wound for their immediate exciting cause, are produced in quite another manner; their source lies in some internal malady. To consider them as mere local affections, and at the same time to treat them only, or almost only, as it were surgically, with topical applications – as the old school have done from the remotest ages – is as absurd as it is pernicious in its results.

§ 188

These affections were considered to be merely topical, and were therefore called local diseases, as if they were maladies exclusively limited to those parts wherein the organism took little or no part, or affections of these particular visible parts of which the rest of the living organism, so to speak, knew nothing. [123]

§ 189

And yet very little reflection will suffice to convince us that no external malady (not occasioned by some important injury from without) can arise, persist or even grow worse without some internal cause, without the co-operation of the whole organism, which must consequently be in a diseased state. It could not make its appearance at all without the consent of the whole of the rest of the health, and without the participation of the rest of the living whole (of the vital force that pervades all the other sensitive and irritable parts of the organism); indeed, it is impossible to conceive its production without the instrumentality of the whole (deranged) life; so intimately are all parts of the organism connected together to form an indivisible whole in sensation and functions. No eruption on the lips, no whitlow can occur without previous and simultaneous internal ill-health.

§ 190

All true medical treatment of a disease on the external parts of the body that has occurred from little or no injury from without must, therefore, be directed against the whole, must effect the annihilation and cure of the general malady by means of internal remedies, if it is wished that the treatment should be judicious, sure, efficacious and radical.

§ 191

This is confirmed in the most unambiguous manner by experience, which shows in all cases that every powerful internal medicine immediately after its ingestion causes important changes in the general health of such a patient, and particularly in the affected external parts (which the ordinary medical school regards as quite isolated), even in a so-called local disease of the most external parts of the body, and the change it produces is most salutary, being the restoration to health of the entire body, along with the disappearance of the external affection (without the aid of any external remedy), provided the internal remedy directed towards the whole state was suitable chosen in a homoeopathic sense.

§ 192

This is best effected when, in the investigation of the case of disease, along with the exact character of the local affection, all the changes, sufferings and symptoms observable in the patient's health, and which may have been previously noticed when no medicines had been used, are taken in conjunction to form a complete picture of the disease before searching among the medicines, whose peculiar pathogenetic effects are known, for a remedy corresponding to the totality of the symptoms, so that the selection may be truly homoeopathic.

§ 193

By means of this medicine, employed only internally (and, if the disease be but of recent origin, often by the very first dose of it), the general morbid state of the body is removed along with the local affection, and the latter is cured at the same time as the former, proving that the local affection depended solely on a disease of the rest of the body, and should only be regarded as an inseparable part of the whole, as one of the most considerable and striking symptoms of the whole disease.

§ 194

It is not useful, either in acute local diseases of recent origin or in local affections that have already existed a long time, to rub in or apply externally to the spot an external remedy, even though it be the specific and, when used internally, salutary by reason of its homoeopathicity, even although it should be at the same time administered internally; for the acute topical affections (e.g., inflammations of the individual parts, erysipelas, etc.), which have not been caused by external injury of proportionate violence, but by dynamic or internal causes, yield most surely to internal remedies homoeopathically adapted to the perceptible state of the health present in the exterior and interior, selected from the general store of proved medicines, [124] and generally without any other aid; but if these diseases do not yield to them completely, and if there still remain in the affected spot and in the whole state, notwithstanding good regimen, a relic of disease which the vital force is not competent to restore to the normal state, then the acute disease was (as not infrequently happens) a product of psora which had hitherto remained latent in the interior, but has now burst forth and is on the point of developing into a palpable chronic disease.

§ 195
In order to effect a radical cure in such cases, which are by no means rare, after the acute state has pretty well subsided, an appropriate antipsoric treatment (as is taught in my work on Chronic Diseases) must then be directed against the symptoms that still remain and the morbid state of health to which the patient was previously subject. In chronic local maladies that are not obviously venereal, the antipsoric internal treatment is, moreover, alone requisite.

§ 196
It might, indeed, seen as though the cure of such diseases would be hastened by employing the medicinal substance which is known to be truly homoeopathic to the totality of the symptoms, not only internally, but also externally, because the action of a medicine applied to the seat of the local affection might effect a more rapid change in it.

§ 197 Fifth Edition
This treatment, however, is quite inadmissible, not only for the local symptoms arising from the miasm of psora, but also and especially for those originating in the miasm of syphilis or sycosis, for the simultaneous local application, along with the internal employment, of the remedy in diseases whose chief symptom is a constant local affection, has this great disadvantage, that, by such a topical application, this chief symptom (local affection) [125] will usually be annihilated sooner than the internal disease, and we shall now be deceived by the semblance of a perfect cure; or at least it will be difficult, and in some cases impossible, to determine, from the premature disappearance of the local symptom, if the general disease is destroyed by the simultaneous employment of the internal medicine.

§ 197 Sixth Edition
This treatment, however, is quite inadmissible, not only for the local symptoms arising from the miasm of psora, but also and especially for those originating in the miasm of syphilis or sycosis, for the simultaneous local application, along with the internal employment, of the remedy in diseases whose chief symptom is a constant local affection, has this great disadvantage, that, by such a topical application, this chief symptom (local affection) [126] will usually be annihilated sooner than the internal disease, and we shall now be deceived by the semblance of a perfect cure; or at least it will be difficult, and in some cases impossible, to determine, from the premature disappearance of the local symptom, if the general disease is destroyed by the simultaneous employment of the internal medicine.

§ 198
The mere topical employment of medicines, that are powerful for cure when given internally, to the local symptoms of chronic miasmatic diseases is for the same reason quite inadmissible; for if the local affection of the chronic disease be only removed locally and in a one-sided manner, the internal treatment indispensable for the complete restoration of the health remains in dubious obscuri-

ty; the chief symptom (the local affection) is gone, and there remain only the other, less distinguishable symptoms, which are less constant and less persistent than the local affection, and frequently not sufficiently peculiar and too slightly characteristic to display after that, a picture of the disease in clear and peculiar outlines.

§ 199

If the remedy perfectly homoeopathic to the disease had not yet been discovered [127] at the time when the local symptoms were destroyed by a corrosive or desiccative external remedy or by the knife, then the case becomes much more difficult on account of the too indefinite (uncharacteristic) and inconstant appearance of the remaining symptoms; for what might have contributed most to determine the selection of the most suitable remedy, and its internal employment until the disease should have been completely annihilated, namely, the external principal symptom, has been removed from our observation.

§ 200 Fifth Edition

Had it still been present to guide the internal treatment, the homoeopathic remedy for the whole disease might have been discovered, and had that been found, the persistence of the local affection during its internal employment would have shown that the cure was not yet completed; but were it cured on its seat, this would be a convincing proof that the disease was completely eradicated, and the desired recovery from the entire disease was fully accomplished – an inestimable, indispensable advantage.

§ 200 Sixth Edition

Had it still been present to guide the internal treatment, the homoeopathic remedy for the whole disease might have been discovered, and had that been found, the persistence of the local affection during its internal employment would have shown that the cure was not yet completed; but were it cured on its seat, this would be a convincing proof that the disease was completely eradicated, and the desired recovery from the entire disease was fully accomplished – an inestimable, indispensable advantage to reach a perfect cure.

§ 201 Fifth Edition

It is evident that man's vital force, when encumbered with a chronic disease which it is unable to overcome by its own powers, adopts the plan of developing a local malady on some external part, solely for this object, that by making and keeping in a diseased state this part which is not indispensable to human life, it may thereby silence the internal disease, which otherwise threatens to destroy the vital organs (and to deprive the patient of life), and that it may thereby, so to speak, transfer the internal disease to the vicarious local affection and, as it were, draw it thither. The presence of the local affection thus silences, for a time, the internal disease, though without being able either to cure it or to diminish it materially. [128] The local affection, however, is never anything else than a part of the general disease, but a part of it increased all in one direction by the organic vital force, and transferred to a less dangerous (external) part of the body, in order to allay the internal ailment. But (as has been said) by this local symptom that silences the internal disease, so far from anything being gained by the vital force towards diminishing or curing the whole malady, the internal disease, on the contrary, continues, in spite of it, gradually to increase and Nature is constrained to enlarge and aggravate the local symptom always more and more, in order that it may still suffice as a substitute for the increased internal disease and may still keep it under. Old ulcers on the legs get worse as long as the internal psora is uncured, the chancre enlarges as long as the internal syphilis remains uncured, just as the general internal disease continues to increase as time goes on.

§ 201 Sixth Edition

It is evident that man's vital force, when encumbered with a chronic disease which it is unable to overcome by its own powers instinctively, adopts the plan of developing a local malady on some external part, solely for this object, that by making and keeping in a diseased state this part which is not indispensable to human life, it may thereby silence the internal disease, which otherwise threatens to destroy the vital organs (and to deprive the patient of life), and that it may thereby, so to speak, transfer the internal disease to the vicarious local affection and, as it were, draw it thither. The presence of the local affection thus silences, for a time, the internal disease, though without being able either to cure it or to diminish it materially. [129] The local affection, however, is never anything else than a part of the general disease, but a part of it increased all in one direction by the organic vital force, and transferred to a less dangerous (external) part of the body, in order to allay the internal ailment. But (as has been said) by this local symptom that silences the internal disease, so far from anything being gained by the vital force towards diminishing or curing the whole malady, the internal disease, on the contrary, continues, in spite of it, gradually to increase and Nature is constrained to enlarge and aggravate the local symptom always more and more, in order that it may still suffice as a substitute for the increased internal disease and may still keep it under. Old ulcers on the legs get worse as long as the internal psora is uncured, the chancre enlarges as long as the internal syphilis remains uncured, the fig warts increased and grow while the sycosis is not cured whereby the latter is rendered more and more difficult to cure, just as the general internal disease continues to increase as time goes on.

§ 202

If the old-school physician should now destroy the local symptom by the topical application of external remedies, under the belief that he thereby cures the whole disease, Nature makes up for its loss by rousing the internal malady and the other symptoms that previously existed in a latent state side by side with the local affection; that is to say, she increases the internal disease. When this occurs it is usual to say, though incorrectly that the local affection has been driven back into the system or upon the nerves by the external remedies.

§ 203

Every external treatment of such local symptoms, the object of which is to remove them from the surface of the body, while the internal miasmatic disease is left uncured, as, for instance, driving off the skin the psoric eruption by all sorts of ointments, burning away the chancre by caustics and destroying the condylomata on their seat by the knife, the ligature or the actual cautery; this pernicious external mode of treatment, hitherto so universally practised, has been the most prolific source of all the innumerable named or unnamed chronic maladies under which mankind groans; it is one of the most criminal procedures the medical world can be guilty of, and yet it has hitherto been the one generally adopted, and taught from the professional chairs as the only one. [130]

§ 204 Fifth Edition

If we deduct all chronic affections, ailments and diseases that depend on a persistent unhealthy mode of living, (§ 77) as also those innumerable medicinal maladies (v. § 74) caused by the irrational, persistent, harassing and pernicious treatment of diseases often only of trivial character by physicians of the old school, all the remainder, without exception, result from the development of these three chronic miasms, internal syphilis, internal sycosis, but chiefly and in infinitely greater proportion, internal psora, each of which was already in possession of the whole organism, and had penetrated it in all directions before the appearance of the primary, vicarious local symptom of each of them (in the case of psora the scabious eruption, in syphilis the chancre or the bubo, and in sycosis the condylomata) that prevented their outburst; and these chronic miasmatic diseases, if deprived of their local symptom, are inevitably destined by mighty Nature sooner or later to become developed and to burst forth, and thereby propagate all the nameless misery, the incredible number of chronic diseases which have plagued mankind for hundreds and thousands of years, none of which would so frequently have come into existence had physicians striven in a rational manner to cure radically and to extinguish in the organism these three miasms by the internal homoeopathic medicines suited for each of them, without employing topical remedies for their external symptoms. (See note to § 282).

§ 204 Sixth Edition

If we deduct all chronic affections, ailments and diseases that depend on a persistent unhealthy mode of living, (§ 77) as also those innumerable medicinal maladies (v. § 74) caused by the irrational, persistent, harassing and pernicious treatment of diseases often only of trivial character by physicians of the old school, most the remainder of chronic diseases result from the development of these three chronic miasms, internal syphilis, internal sycosis, but chiefly and in infinitely greater proportion, internal psora, each of which was already in possession of the whole organism, and had penetrated it in all directions before the appearance of the primary, vicarious local symptom of each of them (in the case of psora the scabious eruption, in syphilis the chancre or the bubo, and in sycosis the condylomata) that prevented their outburst; and these chronic miasmatic diseases, if deprived of their local symptom, are inevitably destined by mighty Nature sooner or later to become developed and to burst forth, and thereby propagate all the nameless misery, the incredible number of chronic diseases which have plagued mankind for hundreds and thousands of years, none of which would so frequently have come into existence had physicians striven in a rational manner to cure radically and to extinguish in the organism these three miasms by the internal homoeopathic medicines suited for each of them, without employing topical remedies for their external symptoms. (See note to § 282).

§ 205 Fifth Edition

The homoeopathic physician never treats one of these primary symptoms of chronic miasms, nor yet one of their secondary affections that result from their further development, by local remedies (neither by those external agents that act dynamically, [131] nor yet by those that act mechanically), but he cures, in cases where the one or the other appears, only the great miasm on which they depend, whereupon its primary, as also its secondary symptoms disappear spontaneously; but as this was not the mode pursued by the old-school practitioners who preceded him in the treatment of the case, the homoeopathic physician generally, alas!, finds that the primary symptoms [132] have already been destroyed by them by means of external remedies, and that he has now to do more with the secondary ones, i.e., the affections resulting from the breaking forth and development of these inherent miasms, but especially with the chronic disease evolved from internal psora, the internal treatment of which, as far as a single physician can elucidate it by many years of reflection, observation and experience, I have endeavored to point out in my work on Chronic Diseases, to which I must refer the reader.

§ 205 Sixth Edition

The homoeopathic physician never treats one of these primary symptoms of chronic miasms, nor yet one of their secondary affections that result from their further development, by local remedies (neither by those external agents that act dynamically, [133] nor yet by those that act mechanically), but he cures, in cases where the one or the other appears, only the great miasm on which they depend, whereupon its primary, as also its secondary symptoms disappear spontaneously; but as this was not the mode pursued by the old-school practitioners who preceded him in the treatment of the case, the homoeopathic physician generally, alas!, finds that the primary symptoms [132] have already been destroyed by them by means of external remedies, and that he has now to do more with the secondary ones, i.e., the affections resulting from the breaking forth and development of these inherent miasms, but especially with the chronic disease evolved from internal psora, the internal treatment of which, as far as a single physician can elucidate it by many years of reflection, observation and experience, I have endeavored to point out in my work on Chronic Diseases, to which I must refer the reader.

§ 206 Fifth Edition

Before commencing the treatment of a chronic disease, it is necessary to make the most careful investigation [134] as to whether the patient has had a venereal infection (or an infection with condylomatous gonorrhoea); for then the treatment must be directed towards this alone, when only the signs of syphilis (or of the rarer condylomatous disease) are present, but this disease is very seldom met with alone nowadays. If such infection have previously occurred, this must also be borne in mind in the treatment of those cases in which psora is present, because in them the latter is complicated with the former, as is always the case when the symptoms are not those of pure syphilis; for when the physician thinks he has a case of old venereal disease before him, he has always, or almost always, to treat a syphilitic affection accompanied mostly by (complicated with) psora, for the internal itch dyscrasia (the psora) is far the most frequent (most certain) fundamental cause of chronic diseases, either united (complicated) with syphilis (or with sycosis), if the latter infections have avowedly occurred; or, as is much more frequently the case, psora is the sole fundamental cause of all other chronic maladies, whatever names they may bear, which are, moreover, so often bungled, increased and disfigured to a monstrous extent by allopathic unskillfulness.

§ 206 Sixth Edition

Before commencing the treatment of a chronic disease, it is necessary to make the most careful investigation [135] as to whether the patient has had a venereal infection (or an infection with condylomatous gonorrhoea); for then the treatment must be directed towards this alone, when only the signs of syphilis (or of the rarer condylomatous disease) are present, but this disease is very seldom met with alone nowadays. If such infection have previously occurred, this must also be borne in mind in the treatment of those cases in which psora is present, because in them the latter is complicated with the former, as is always the case when the symptoms are not those of pure syphilis; for when the physician thinks he has a case of old venereal disease before him, he has always, or almost always, to treat a syphilitic affection accompanied mostly by (complicated with) psora, for the internal itch dyscrasia (the psora) is far the most frequent fundamental cause of chronic diseases. At times, both miasms may be complicated also with sycosis in chronically diseased organisms, or, as is much more frequently the case, psora is the sole fundamental cause of all other chronic maladies, whatever names they may bear, which are, moreover, so often bungled, increased and disfigured to a monstrous extent by allopathic unskillfulness.

§ 207

When the above information has been gained, it still remains for the homoeopathic physician to ascertain what kinds of allopathic treatment had up to that date been adopted for the chronic disease, what perturbing medicines had been chiefly and most frequently employed, also what mineral baths had been used and what effects these had produced, in order to understand in some measure the degeneration of the disease from its original state, and, where possible, to correct in part these pernicious artificial operations, or to enable him to avoid the employment of medicines that have already been improperly used.

§ 208

The age of the patient, his mode of living and diet, his occupation, his domestic position, his social relation and so forth, must next be taken into consideration, in order to ascertain whether these things have tended to increase his malady, or in how far they may favor or hinder the treatment. In like manner the state of his disposition and mind must be attended to, to learn whether that presents any obstacles to the treatment, or requires to be directed encouraged or modified.

§ 209

After this is done, the physician should endeavor in repeated conversations with the patient to trace the picture of his disease as completely as possible, according to the directions given above, in order to be able to elucidate the most striking and peculiar (characteristic) symptoms, in accordance with which he selects the first antipsoric or other remedy having the greatest symptomatic resemblance, for the commencement of the treatment, and so forth.

§ 210

Of psoric origin are almost all those diseases that I have above termed one-sided, which appear to be more difficult to cure in consequence of this one-sidedness, all their other morbid symptoms disappearing, as it were, before the single, great, prominent symptom. Of this character are what are termed mental diseases. They do not, however, constitute a class of disease the condition of the disposition and mind is always altered; [136] and in all cases of disease we are called on to cure the state of the patient's disposition is to be particularly noted, along with the totality of the symptoms, if we would trace an accurate picture of the disease, in order to be able therefrom to treat it homoeopathically with success.

§ 211

This holds good to such an extent, that the state of the disposition of the patient often chiefly determines the selection of the homoeopathic remedy, as being a decidedly characteristic symptom which can least of all remain concealed from the accurately observing physician.

§ 212

The Creator of therapeutic agents has also had particular regard to this main feature of all diseases, the altered state of the disposition and mind, for there is no powerful medicinal substance in the world which does not very notably alter the state of the disposition and mind in the healthy individual who tests it, and every medicine does so in a different manner.

§ 213

We shall, therefore, never be able to cure conformably to nature – that is to say, homoeopathically – if we do not, in every case of disease, even in such as are acute, observe, along with the other symptoms, those relating to the changes in the state of the mind and disposition, and if we do not select, for the patient's relief, from among the medicines a disease-force which, in addition to the similarity of its other symptoms to those of the disease, is also capable of producing a similar state of the disposition and mind. [137]

§ 214

The instructions I have to give relative to the cure of mental diseases may be confined to a very few remarks, as they are to be cured in the same way as all other diseases, namely, by a remedy which shows, by the symptoms it causes in the body and mind of a healthy individual, a power of producing a morbid state as similar as possible to the case of disease before us, and in no other way can they be cured.

§ 215

Almost all the so-called mental and emotional diseases are nothing more than corporeal diseases in which the symptom of derangement of the mind and disposition peculiar to each of them is increased, while the corporeal symptoms decline (more or less rapidly), till it a length attains the most striking one-sidedness, almost as though it were a local disease in the invisible subtle organ of the mind or disposition.

§ 216

The cases are not rare in which a so-called corporeal disease that threatens to be fatal – a suppuration of the lungs, or the deterioration of some other important viscus, or some other disease of acute character, e.g., in childbed, etc. – becomes transformed into insanity, into a kind of melancholia or into mania by a rapid increase of the psychical symptoms that were previously present, whereupon the corporeal symptoms lose all their danger; these latter improve almost to perfect health, or rather they decrease to such a degree that their obscured presence can only be detected by the observation of a physician gifted with perseverance and penetration. In this manner they become transformed into a one-sided and, as it were, a local disease, in which the symptom of the mental disturbance, which was at first but slight, increases so as to be the chief symptom, and in a great measure occupies the place of the other (corporeal) symptoms, whose intensity it subdues in a palliative manner, so that, in short, the affections of the grosser corporeal organs become, as it were, transferred and conducted to the almost spiritual, mental and emotional organs, which the anatomist has never yet and never will reach with his scalpel.

§ 217

In these diseases we must be very careful to make ourselves acquainted with the whole of the phenomena, both those belonging to the corporeal symptoms, and also, and indeed particularly, those appertaining to the accurate apprehension of the precise character of the chief symptom, of the peculiar and always predominating state of the mind and disposition, in order to discover, for the purpose of extinguishing the entire disease, among the remedies whose pure effects are known, a homoeopathic medicinal pathogenetic force – that is to say, a remedy which in its list of symptoms displays, with the greatest possible similarity, not only the corporeal morbid symptoms present in the case of disease before us, but also especially this mental and emotional state.

§ 218

To this collection of symptoms belongs in the first place to accurate description of all the phenomena of the previous so-called corporeal disease, before it degenerated into a one-sided increase of the physical symptom, and became a disease of the mind and disposition. This may be learned from the report of the patient's friends.

§ 219

A comparison of these previous symptoms of the corporeal disease with the traces of them that still remain, though they have become less perceptible (but which even now sometimes become prominent, when a lucid interval and a transient alleviation of the psychical disease occurs), will serve to prove them to be still present, though obscured.

§ 220

By adding to this the state of the mind and disposition accurately observed by the patient's friends and by the physician himself, we have thus constructed the complete picture of the disease, for which in order to effect the homoeopathic cure of the disease, a medicine capable of producing strikingly similar symptoms, and especially an analogous disorder of the mind, must be sought for among the antipsoric remedies, if the physical disease have already lasted some time.

§ 221

If, however, insanity or mania (caused by fright, vexation, the abuse of spirituous liquors, etc.) have suddenly broken out as an acute disease in the patient's ordinary calm state, although it almost always arises from internal psora, like a flame bursting forth from it, yet when it occurs in this acute manner it should not be immediately treated with antipsoric, but in the first place with remedies indicated for it out of the order class of proved medicaments (e.g., aconite, belladonna, stramonium, hyoscyamus, mercury, etc.) in highly potentized, minute, homoeopathic doses, in order to subdue it so far that the psora shall for the time revert to its former latent state, wherein the patient appears as if quite well.

§ 222

But such a patient, who has recovered from an acute mental or emotional disease by the use of these non-antipsoric medicines, should never be regarded as cured; on the contrary, no time should be lost in attempting to free him completely, [138] by means of a prolonged antipsoric treatment, from the chronic miasm of the psora, which, it is true, has now become once more latent but is quite ready to break out anew; if this be done, there is no fear of another similar attack, if he attend faithfully to the diet and regimen prescribed for him.

§ 223

But if the antipsoric treatment be omitted, then we may almost assuredly expect, from a much slighter cause than brought on the first attack of the insanity, the speedy occurrence of a new and more lasting the severe fit, during which the psora usually develops itself completely, and passes into either a periodic or continued mental derangement, which is then more difficult to be cured by antipsorics.

§ 224

If the mental disease be not quite developed, and if it be still somewhat doubtful whether it really arose from a corporeal affection, or did not rather result from faults of education, bad practices, corrupt morals, neglect of the mind, superstition or ignorance; the mode of deciding this point will be, that if it proceed from one or other of the latter causes it will diminish and be improved by sensible friendly exhortations, consolatory arguments, serious representations and sensible advice, whereas a real moral or mental malady, depending on bodily disease, would be speedily aggravated by such a course, the melancholic would become still more dejected, querulous, inconsolable and reserved, the spiteful maniac would thereby become still more exasperated, and the chattering fool would become manifestly more foolish. [139]

§ 225

There are, however, as has just been stated, certainly a few emotional diseases which have not merely been developed into that form out of corporeal diseases, but which, in an inverse manner, the body being but slightly indisposed, originate and are kept up by emotional causes, such as continued anxiety, worry, vexation, wrongs and the frequent occurrence of great fear and fright. This kind of emotional diseases in time destroys the corporeal health, often to a great degree.

§ 226

It is only such emotional diseases as these, which were first engendered and subsequently kept up by the mind itself, that, while they are yet recent and before they have made very great inroads on the corporeal state, may, by means of psychical remedies, such as a display of confidence, friendly exhortations, sensible advice, and often by a well-disguised deception, be rapidly changed into a healthy state of the mind (and with appropriate diet and regimen, seemingly into a healthy state of the body also.)

§ 227

But the fundamental cause in these cases also is a psoric miasm, which was only not yet quite near its full development, and for security's sake, the seemingly cured patient should be subjected to a radical, antipsoric treatment, in order that he may not again, as might easily occur, fall into a similar state of mental disease.

§ 228

In mental and emotional diseases resulting from corporeal maladies, which can only be cured by homoeopathic antipsoric medicine conjoined with carefully regulated mode of life, an appropriate psychical behavior towards the patient on the part of those about him and of the physician must be scrupulously observed, by way of an auxiliary mental regimen. To furious mania we must oppose clam intrepidity and cool, firm resolution – to doleful, querulous lamentation, a mute display of commiseration in looks and gestures – to senseless chattering, a silence not wholly inattentive – to disgusting and abominable conduct and to conversation of a similar character, total inattention. We must merely endeavor to prevent the destruction and injury of surrounding objects, without reproaching the patient for his acts, and everything must be arranged in such a way that the necessity for any corporeal punishments and tortures [140] whatever may be avoided. This is so much the more easily effected, because in the administration of the medicine – the only circumstance in which the employment of coercion could be justified – in the homoeopathic system the small doses of the appropriate medicine never offend the taste, and may consequently be given to the patient without his knowledge in his drink, so that all compulsion is unnecessary.

§ 229

On the other hand, contradiction, eager explanations, rude corrections and invectives, as also weak, timorous yielding, are quite out of place with such patients; they are equally pernicious modes of treating mental and emotional maladies. But such patients are most of all exasperated and their complaint aggravated by contumely, fraud, and deceptions that they can detect. The physician and keeper must always pretend to believe them to be possessed of reason.

All kinds of external disturbing influences on their senses and disposition should be if possible removed; there are no amusements for their clouded spirit, no salutary distractions, no means of instruction, no soothing effects from conversation, books or other things for the soul that pines or frets in the chains of the diseased body, no invigoration for it, but the care; it is only when the bodily health is changed for the better that tranquillity and comfort again beam upon their mind. [141]

§ 230

If the antipsoric remedies selected for each particular case of mental or emotional disease (there are incredibly numerous varieties of them) be quite homoeopathically suited for the faithfully traced picture of the morbid state, which, if there be a sufficient number of this kind of medicines known in respect of their pure effects, is ascertained by an indefatigable search for the most appropriate homoeopathic remedy all the more easily, as the emotional and mental state, constituting the principal symptom of such a patient, is so unmistakably perceptible, – then the most striking improvement in no very long time, which could not be brought about by physicking the patient to death with the largest oft – repeated doses of all other unsuitable (allopathic) medicines. Indeed, I can confidently assert, from great experience, that the vast superiority of the homoeopathic system over all other conceivable methods of the treatment is nowhere displayed in a more triumphant light than in mental and emotional diseases of long standing, which originally sprang from corporeal maladies or were developed simultaneously with them.

§ 231
The intermittent disease deserve a special consideration, as well those that recur at certain periods – like the great number of intermittent fevers, and the apparently non-febrile affections that recur at intervals like intermittent fevers – as also those in which certain morbid states alternate at uncertain intervals with morbid states of a different kind.

§ 232
These latter, alternating diseases, are also very numerous, [142] but all belong to the class of chronic diseases; they are generally a manifestation of developed psora alone, sometimes, but seldom, complicated with a syphilitic miasm, and therefore in the former case may be cured by antipsoric medicines; in the latter, however, in alternation with antisyphilitics as taught in my work on the Chronic Diseases.

§ 233
The typical intermittent disease are those where a morbid state of unvarying character returns at a tolerably fixed period, while the patient is apparently in good health, and takes its departure at an equally fixed period; this is observed in those apparently non-febrile morbid states that come and go in a periodical manner (at certain times), as well as in those of a febrile character, to wit, the numerous varieties of intermittent fevers.

§ 234
Those apparently non-febrile, typical, periodically recurring morbid states just alluded to observed in one single patient at a time (they do not usually appear sporadically or epidemically) always belong to the chronic diseases, mostly to those that are purely psoric, are but seldom complicated with syphilis, and are successfully treated by the same means; yet it is sometimes necessary to employ as an intermediate remedy a small dose of a potentized solution of cinchona bark, in order to extinguish completely their intermittent type.

§ 235
With regard to the intermittent fevers, [143] that prevail sporadically or epidemically (not those endemically located in marshy districts), we often find every paroxysm likewise composed of two opposite alternating states (cold, heat – heat, cold), more frequently still of three (cold, heat, sweat). Therefore the remedy selected for them from the general class of proved (common, not antipsoric) medicines must either (and remedies of this sort are the surest) be able likewise to produce in the healthy body two (or all three) similar alternating states, or else must correspond by similarity of symptoms, in the most homoeopathic manner possible, to the strongest, best marked, and most peculiar alternating state (either to the cold stage, or to the hot stage, or to the sweating state, each with its accessory symptoms, according as the one or other alternating state is the strongest and most peculiar); but the symptoms of the patient's health during the intervals when he is free from fever must be the chief guide to the most appropriate homoeopathic remedy. [144]

§ 236

The most appropriate and efficacious time for administering the medicine in these cases is immediately or very soon after the termination of the paroxysm, as soon as the patient has in some degree recovered from its effects; it has then time to effect all the changes in the organism requisite for the restoration of health, without any great disturbance or violent commotion; whereas the action of a medicine, be it ever so specifically appropriate, if given immediately before the paroxysm, coincides with the natural recurrence of the disease and causes such a reaction in the organism, such a violent contention, that an attack of that nature produces at the very least a great loss of strength, if it do not endanger life. [145] But if the medicine be given immediately after the termination of the fit, that is to say, at the period when the apyretic interval has commenced and a long time before there are any preparations for the next paroxysm, then the vital force of the organism is in the best possible condition to allow itself to be quietly altered by the remedy, and thus restored to the healthy state.

§ 237

But if the stage of apyrexia be very short, as happens in some very bad fevers, or if it be disturbed by some of the after sufferings of the previous paroxysm, the dose of the homoeopathic medicine should be administered when the perspiration begins to abate, or the other subsequent phenomena of the expiring paroxysm begin to diminish.

§ 238 Fifth Edition

It is only when the suitable medicine has with a single dose destroyed several fits and manifest health and ensued, but after some time indications of a new paroxysm appear, only then can and must the same medicine be given again, provided always the totality of the symptoms is still the same. This recurrence of the same fever after an interval of health is, however, only possible when the noxious influence that first excited the intermittent fever still continues to act upon the convalescent, as happens in marshy districts; in which case a permanent cure is often only possible by the removal of this exciting cause (as, for instance, a residence in a mountainous country if the case was one of marsh intermittent fever).

§ 238 Sixth Edition

Not infrequently, the suitable medicine has with a single dose destroyed several attacks and brought about the return of health, but in the majority of cases, another dose must be administered after such attack. Better still, however, when the character of the symptoms has not changed, doses of the same medicine given according to the newer discovery of repetition of doses (see note to § 270), may be given without difficulty in dynamizing each successive dose with 10-12 successions of the vial containing the medicinal substance. Nevertheless, there are at times cases, though seldom, where the intermittent fever returns after several days' well being. This return of the same fever after a healthy interval is only possible when the noxious principle that first caused the fever, is still acting upon the convalescent, as is the case in marshy regions. Here a permanent restoration can often take place only by getting away from this causative factor, as is possible by seeking a mountainous retreat, if the cause was a marshy fever.

§ 239

As almost every medicine causes in its pure action a special, peculiar fever and even a kind of intermittent fever with its alternating states, differing from all other fevers that are caused by other medicines, homoeopathic remedies may be found in the extensive domain of medicines for all the numerous varieties of natural intermittent fevers and, for a great many of such fevers, even in the moderate collection of medicines already proved on the healthy individual.

§ 240
But if the remedy found to be the homoeopathic specific for a prevalent epidemic of intermittent fever do not effect a perfect cure in some one or other patient, if it be not the influence of a marshy district that prevents the cure, it must always be the psoric miasm in the background, in which case antipsoric medicines must be employed until complete relief is obtained.

§ 241
Epidemics of intermittent fever, in situations where none are endemic, are of the nature of chronic diseases, composed of single acute paroxysms; each single epidemic is of a peculiar, uniform character common to all the individuals attacked, and when this character is found in the totality of the symptoms common to all, it guides us to the discovery of the homoeopathic (specific) remedy suitable for all the cases, which is almost universally serviceable in those patients who enjoyed tolerable health before the occurrence of the epidemic, that is to say, who were not chronic sufferers from developed psora.

§ 242
If, however, in such an epidemic intermittent fever the first paroxysms have been left uncured, or if the patients have been weakened by improper allopathic treatment; then the inherent psora that exists, alas! in so many persons, although in a latent state, becomes developed, takes on the type of the intermittent fever, and to all appearance continues to play the part of the epidemic intermittent fever, so that the medicine, which would have been useful in the first paroxysms (rarely an antipsoric), is now no longer suitable and cannot be of any service. We have now to do with a psoric intermittent fever only, and this will generally be subdued by minute and rarely repeated doses of sulphur or hepar sulphuris in a high potency.

§ 243
In those often very pernicious intermittent fevers which attack a single person, not residing in a marshy district, we must also at first, as in the case of acute diseases generally, which they resemble in respect to their psoric origin, employ for some days, to render what service it may, a homoeopathic remedy selected for the special case from the other class of proved (not antipsoric) medicines; but if, notwithstanding this procedure, the recovery is deferred, we know that we have psora on the point of its development, and that in this case antipsoric medicines alone can effect a radical cure.

§ 244 Fifth Edition
The intermittent fevers endemic in marshy districts and tracts of country frequently exposed to inundations, give a great deal of work to physicians of the old school, and yet a healthy man may in his youth become habituated even to marshy districts and remain in good health, provided he preserves a faultless regimen and his system is not lowered by want, fatigue or pernicious passions. The intermittent fevers endemic there would at the most only attack him on his first arrival; but one or two very small doses of a highly potentized solution of

cinchona bark would, conjointly with the well-regulated mode of living just alluded to, speedily free him from the disease. But persons who, while taking sufficient corporeal exercise and pursuing a healthy system of intellectual occupations and bodily regimen, cannot be cured of marsh intermittent fever by one or a few of such small doses of cinchona – in such persons psora, striving to develop itself, always lies at the root of their malady, and their intermittent fever cannot be cured in the marshy district without antipsoric treatment. [146] It sometimes happens that when these patients exchange, without delay, the marshy district for one that is dry and mountainous, recovery apparently ensues (the fever leaves them) if they be not yet deeply sunk in disease, that is to say, if the psora was not completely developed in them and can consequently return to its latent state; but they will never regain perfect health without antipsoric treatment.

§ 244 Sixth Edition
The intermittent fevers endemic in marshy districts and tracts of country frequently exposed to inundations, give a great deal of work to physicians of the old school, and yet a healthy man may in his youth become habituated even to marshy districts and remain in good health, provided he preserves a faultless regimen and his system is not lowered by want, fatigue or pernicious passions. The intermittent fevers endemic there would at the most only attack him on his first arrival; but one or two very small doses of a highly potentized solution of cinchona bark would, conjointly with the well-regulated mode of living just alluded to, speedily free him from the disease. But persons who, while taking sufficient corporeal exercise and pursuing a healthy system of intellectual occupations and bodily regimen, cannot be cured of marsh intermittent fever by one or a few of such small doses of cinchona – in such persons psora, striving to develop itself, always lies at the root of their malady, and their intermittent fever cannot be cured in the marshy district without antipsoric treatment. [147] It sometimes happens that when these patients exchange, without delay, the marshy district for one that is dry and mountainous, recovery apparently ensues (the fever leaves them) if they be not yet deeply sunk in disease, that is to say, if the psora was not completely developed in them and can consequently return to its latent state; but they will never regain perfect health without antipsoric treatment.

§ 245 Fifth Edition
Having thus seen what attention should, in the homoeopathic treatment, be paid to the chief varieties of diseases and to the peculiar circumstances connected with them, we now pass on to what we have to say respecting the remedies and the mode of employing them, together with the diet and regimen to be observed during their use.

§ 245 Sixth Edition
Having thus seen what attention should, in the homoeopathic treatment, be paid to the chief varieties of diseases and to the peculiar circumstances connected with them, we now pass on to what we have to say respecting the remedies and the mode of employing them, together with the diet and regimen to be observed during their use.

Every perceptibly progressive and strikingly increasing amelioration in a transient (acute) or persistent (chronic) disease, is a condition which, as long as it lasts, completely precludes every repetition of the administration of any medicine whatsoever, because all the good the medicine taken continues to effect is new hastening towards its completion. Every new dose of any medicine whatsoever, even of the one last administered, that has hitherto shown itself to be salutary, would in this case disturb the work of amelioration.

§ 246 Fifth Edition

On the other hand, the slowly progressive amelioration consequent on a very minute dose, whose selection has been accurately homoeopathic, when it has met with no hindrance to the duration of its action, sometimes accomplishes all the good the remedy in question is capable from its nature of performing in a given case, in periods of forty, fifty or a hundred days. This is, however, but rarely the case; and besides, it must be a matter of great importance to the physician as well as to the patient that were it possible, this period should be diminished to one-half, one-quarter, and even still less, so that a much more rapid cure might be obtained. And this may be very happily affected, as recent and oft-repeated observations have shown, under three conditions: firstly, if the medicine selected with the utmost care was perfectly homoeopathic; secondly, if it was given in the minutest dose, so as to produce the least possible excitation of the vital force, and yet sufficient to effect the necessary change in it; and thirdly, if this minutest yet powerful dose of the best selected medicine be repeated at suitable intervals, [148] which experience shall have pronounced to be the best adapted for accelerating the cure to the utmost extent, yet without the vital force, which it is sought to influence to the production of a similar medicinal disease, being able to feel itself excited and roused to adverse reactions.

§ 246 Sixth Edition

Every perceptibly progressive and strikingly increasing amelioration during treatment is a condition which, as long as it lasts, completely precludes every repetition of the administration of any medicine whatsoever, because all the good the medicine taken continues to effect is now hastening towards its completion. This is not infrequently the cause in acute diseases, but in more chronic diseases, on the other hand, a single dose of an appropriately selected homoeopathic remedy will at times complete even with but slowly progressive improvement and give the help which such a remedy in such a case can accomplish naturally within 40, 50, 60, 100 days. This is, however, but rarely the case; and besides, it must be a matter of great importance to the physician as well as to the patient that were it possible, this period should be diminished to one-half, one-quarter, and even still less, so that a much more rapid cure might be obtained. And this may be very happily affected, as recent and oft-repeated observations have taught me under the following conditions: firstly, if the medicine selected with the utmost care was perfectly homoeopathic; secondly, if it is highly potentized, dissolved in water and given in proper small dose that experience has taught as the most suitable in definite intervals for the quickest accomplishment of the cure but with the precaution, that the degree of every dose deviate somewhat from the preceding and following in order that the vital principle which is to be altered to a similar medicinal disease be not aroused to untoward reactions and revolt as is always the case [148b] with unmodified and especially rapidly repeated doses.

§ 247 Fifth Edition

Under these conditions, the smallest doses of the best selected homoeopathic medicine may be repeated with the best, often with incredible results, at intervals of fourteen, twelve, ten, eight, seven days, and, where rapidity is requisite, in chronic diseases resembling cases of acute disease, at still shorter intervals, but in acute diseases at very much shorter periods – every twenty – four, twelve, eight, four hours, in the very acutest every hour, up to as often as every five minutes, – in ever case in proportion to the more or less rapid course of the diseases and of the action of the medicine employed, as is more distinctly explained in the last note.

§ 247 Sixth Edition
It is impractical to repeat the same unchanged dose of a remedy once, not to mention its frequent repetition (and at short intervals in order not to delay the cure). The vital principle does not accept such unchanged doses without resistance, that is, without other symptoms of the medicine to manifest themselves than those similar to the disease to be cured, because the former dose has already accomplished the expected change in the vital principle and a second dynamically wholly similar, unchanged dose of the same medicine no longer finds, therefore, the same conditions of the vital force. The patient may indeed be made sick in another way by receiving other such unchanged doses, even sicker than he was, for now only those symptoms of the given remedy remain active which were not homoeopathic to the original disease, hence no step towards cure can follow, only a true aggravation of the condition of the patient. But if the succeeding dose is changed slightly every time, namely potentized somewhat higher (§§ 269-270) then the vital principle may be altered without difficulty by the same medicine (the sensation of natural disease diminishing) and thus the cure brought nearer. [149]

§ 248 Fifth Edition
The dose of the same medicine may be repeated several times according to circumstances, but only so long as until either recovery ensues, or the same remedy ceases to do good and the rest of the disease, presenting a different group of symptoms, demands a different homoeopathic remedy.

§ 248 Sixth Edition
For this purpose, we potentize anew the medicinal solution [150] (with perhaps 8, 10, 12 successions) from which we give the patient one or (increasingly) several teaspoonful doses, in long lasting diseases daily or every second day, in acute diseases every two to six hours and in very urgent cases every hour or oftener. Thus in chronic diseases, every correctly chosen homoeopathic medicine, even those whose action is of long duration, may be repeated daily for months with ever increasing success. If the solution is used up (in seven to fifteen days) it is necessary to add to the next solution of the same medicine if still indicated one or (though rarely) several pellets of a higher potency with which we continue so long as the patient experiences continued improvement without encountering one or another complaint that he never had before in his life. For if this happens, if the balance of the disease appears in a group of altered symptoms then another, one more homoeopathically related medicine must be chosen in place of the last and administered in the same repeated doses, mindful, however, of modifying the solution of every dose with thorough vigorous successions, thus

changing its degree of potency and increasing it somewhat. On the other hand, should there appear during almost daily repetition of the well indicated homoeopathic remedy, towards the end of the treatment of a chronic disease, so-called (§ 161) homoeopathic aggravations by which the balance of the morbid symptoms seem to again increase somewhat (the medicinal disease, similar to the original, now alone persistently manifests itself). The doses in that case must then be reduced still further and repeated in longer intervals and possibly stopped several days, in order to see if the convalescence need no further medicinal aid. The apparent symptoms (Schein – Symptome) caused by the excess of the homoeopathic medicine will soon disappear and leave undisturbed health in its wake. If only a small vial say a dram of dilute alcohol is used in the treatment, in which is contained and dissolved through succussion one globule of the medicine which is to be used by olfaction every two, three or four days, this also must be thoroughly succussed eight to ten times before each olfaction.

§ 249
Every medicine prescribed for a case of disease which, in the course of its action, produces new and troublesome symptoms not appertaining to the disease to be cured, is not capable of effecting real improvement, [151] and cannot be considered as homoeopathically selected; it must, therefore, either, if the aggravation be considerable, be first partially neutralized as soon as possible by an antidote before giving the next remedy chosen more accurately according to similarity of action; or if the troublesome symptoms be not very violent, the next remedy must be given immediately, in order to take the place of the improperly selected one. [152]

§ 250
When, to the observant practitioner who accurately investigates the state of the disease, it is evident, in urgent cases after the lapse of only six, eight or twelve hours, that he has made a bad selection in the medicine last given, in that the patient's state is growing perceptibly, however slightly, worse from hour to hour, by the occurrence of new symptoms and sufferings, it is not only allowable for him, but it is his duty to remedy his mistake, by the selection and administration of a homoeopathic medicine not merely tolerably suitable, but the most appropriate possible for the existing state of the disease (§ 167).

§251
There are some medicines (e.g., ignatia, also bryonia and rhus, and sometimes belladonna) whose power of altering man's health consists chiefly in alternating actions – a kind of primary-action symptoms that are in part opposed to each other. Should the practitioner find, on prescribing one of these, selected on strict homoeopathic principles, that no improvement follows, he will in most cases soon effect his object by giving (in acute diseases, even within a few hours) a fresh and equally small dose of the same medicine. [153]

§ 252
But should we find, during the employment of the other medicines in chronic (psoric) diseases, that the best selected homoeopathic (antipsoric) medicine in the suitable (minutest) dose does not effect an improvement, this is a sure sign that the cause that keeps up the disease still persists, and that there is some cir-

cumstances in the mode of life of the patient or in the situation in which he is placed, that must be removed in order that a permanent cure may ensue.

§ 253
Among the signs that, in all diseases, especially in such as are of an acute nature, inform us of a slight commencement of amelioration or aggravation that is not perceptible to every one, the state of mind and the whole demeanor of the patient are the most certain and instructive. In the case of ever so slight an improvement we observe a greater degree of comfort, increased calmness and freedom of the mind, higher spirits – a kind of return of the natural state. In the case of ever so small a commencement of aggravation we have, on the contrary, the exact opposite of this: a constrained helpless, pitiable state of the disposition, of the mind, of the whole demeanor, and of all gestures, postures and actions, which may be easily perceived on close observation, but cannot be described in words. [154]

§ 254
The other new or increased symptoms or, on the contrary, the diminution of the original ones without any addition of new ones, will soon dispel all doubts from the mind of the attentively observing and investigating practitioner with regard to the aggravation or amelioration; though there are among patients persons who are either incapable of giving an account of this amelioration or aggravation, or are unwilling to confess it.

§ 255 Fifth Edition
But even with such individuals we may convince ourselves on this point by going with them through all the symptoms enumerated in our notes of the disease one by one, and finding that they complain of no new unusual symptoms in addition to these, and that none of the old symptoms are worse. If this be the case, and if an improvement in the disposition and mind have already been observed, the medicine must have effected positive diminution of the disease, or, if sufficient time have not yet elapsed for this, it will soon effect it. Now, supposing the remedy is perfectly appropriate, if the improvement delay too long in making its appearance, this depends either on some error of conduct on the part of the patient, or on the homoeopathic aggravation produced by medicine lasting too long (§ 157), consequently on the dose not being small enough.

§ 255 Sixth Edition
But even with such individuals we may convince ourselves on this point by going with them through all the symptoms enumerated in our notes of the disease one by one, and finding that they complain of no new unusual symptoms in addition to these, and that none of the old symptoms are worse. If this be the case, and if an improvement in the disposition and mind have already been observed, the medicine must have effected positive diminution of the disease, or, if sufficient time have not yet elapsed for this, it will soon effect it. Now, supposing the remedy is perfectly appropriate, if the improvement delay too long in making its appearance, this depends either on some error of conduct on the part of the patient, or on other interfering circumstances.

§ 256 Fifth Edition
On the other hand, if the patient mention the occurrence of some fresh accidents and symptoms of importance – signs that the medicine chosen has not been

strictly homoeopathic – even though he should good-naturedly assure us that he feels better, we must not believe this assurance, but regard his state as aggravated as it will soon be perfectly apparent it is.

§ 256 Sixth Edition
On the other hand, if the patient mention the occurrence of some fresh accidents and symptoms of importance – signs that the medicine chosen has not been strictly homoeopathic – even though he should good-naturedly assure us that he feels better, as is not infrequently the case in phthisical patients with lung abscess, we must not believe this assurance, but regard his state as aggravated as it will soon be perfectly apparent it is.

§ 257
The true physician will take care to avoid making favorite remedies of medicines, the employment of which he has, by chance, perhaps found often useful, and which he has had opportunities of using with good effect. If he do so, some remedies or rarer use, which would have been more homoeopathically suitable, consequently more serviceable, will often be neglected.

§ 258
The true practitioner, moreover, will not in his practice with mistrustful weakness neglect the employment of those remedies that he may now and then have employed with bad effects, owing to an erroneous selection (from his own fault, therefore), or avoid them for other (false) reasons, as that they were unhomoeopathic for the case of disease before him; he must bear in mind the truth, that of medicinal agents that one alone invariably deserves the preference in every case of disease which correspond most accurately by similarity to the totality of the characteristic symptoms, and that no paltry prejudices should interfere with this serious choice.

§ 259
Considering the minuteness of the doses necessary and proper in homoeopathic treatment, we can easily understand that during the treatment everything must be removed from the diet and regimen which can have any medicinal action, in order that the small dose may not be overwhelmed and extinguished or disturbed by any foreign medicinal irritant. [155]

§ 260 Fifth Edition
Hence the careful investigation into such obstacles to cure is so much the more necessary in the case of patients affected by chronic diseases, as their diseases are usually aggravated by such noxious influences and other disease-causing errors in the diet and regimen, which often pass unnoticed. [156]

§ 260 Sixth Edition
Hence the careful investigation into such obstacles to cure is so much the more necessary in the case of patients affected by chronic diseases, as their diseases are usually aggravated by such noxious influences and other disease-causing errors in the diet and regimen, which often pass unnoticed. [157]

§ 261
The most appropriate regimen during the employment of medicine in chronic diseases consists in the removal of such obstacles to recovery, and in supplying where necessary the reverse: innocent moral and intellectual recreation, active

exercise in the open air in almost all kinds of weather (daily walks, slight manual labor), suitable, nutritious, unmedicinal food and drink, etc.

§ 262
In acute diseases, on the other hand – except in cases of mental alienation – the subtle, unerring internal sense of the awakened life-preserving faculty determines so clearly and precisely, that the physician only requires to counsel the friends and attendants to put no obstacles in the way of this voice of nature by refusing anything the patient urgently desires in the way of food, or by trying to persuade him to partake of anything injurious.

§ 263
The desire of the patient affected by an acute disease with regard to food and drink is certainly chiefly for things that give palliative relief: they are, however, not strictly speaking of a medicinal character, and merely supply a sort of want. The slight hindrances that the gratification of this desire, within moderate bounds, could oppose to the radical removal of the disease [158] will be amply counteracted and overcome by the power of the homoeopathically suited medicine and the vital force set free by it, as also by the refreshment that follows from taking what has been so ardently longed for. In like manner, in acute diseases the temperature of the room and the heat or coolness of the bed-coverings must also be arranged entirely in conformity with the patients' wish. He must be kept free from all over-exertion of mind and exciting emotions.

§ 264
The true physician must be provided with genuine medicines of unimpaired strength, so that he may be able to rely upon their therapeutic powers; he must be able, himself, to judge of their genuineness.

§ 265 Fifth Edition
It should be a matter of conscience with him to be thoroughly convinced in every case that the patient always takes the right medicine.

§ 265 Sixth Edition
It should be a matter of conscience with him to be thoroughly convinced in every case that the patient always takes the right medicine and therefore he must give the patient the correctly chosen medicine prepared, moreover, by himself.

§ 266
Substances belonging to the animal and vegetable kingdoms possess their medicinal qualities most perfectly in their raw state. [159]

§ 267
We gain possession of the powers of indigenous plants and of such as may be had in a fresh state in the most complete and certain manner by mixing their freshly expressed juice immediately with equal parts of spirits of wine of a strength sufficient to burn in a lamp. After this has stood a day and a night in a close stoppered bottle and deposited the fibrinous and albuminous matters, the clear superincumbent fluid is then to be decanted off for medicinal use. [160] All fermentation of the vegetable juice will be at once checked by the spirits of wine mixed with it and rendered impossible for the future, and the entire medicinal power of the vegetable juice is thus retained (perfect and uninjured) for ever by keeping the preparation in well-corked bottles and excluded from the sun's light. [161]

§ 268

The other exotic plants, barks, seeds and roots that cannot be obtained in the fresh state the sensible practitioner will never take in the pulverized form on trust, but will first convince himself of their genuineness in their crude, entire state before making any employment of them. [162]

§ 269 Fifth Edition

The homoeopathic system of medicine develops for its use, to a hitherto unheard-of degree, the spirit-like medicinal powers of the crude substances by means of a process peculiar to it and which has hitherto never been tried, whereby only they all become penetratingly efficacious [263] and remedial, even those that in the crude state give no evidence of the slightest medicinal power on the human body.

§ 269 Sixth Edition

The homoeopathic system of medicine develops for its special use, to a hitherto unheard-of degree, the inner medicinal powers of the crude substances by means of a process peculiar to it and which has hitherto never been tried, whereby only they all become immeasurably and penetratingly efficacious [163] and remedial, even those that in the crude state give no evidence of the slightest medicinal power on the human body.

This remarkable change in the qualities of natural bodies develops the latent, hitherto unperceived, as if slumbering [164] hidden, dynamic (§ 11) powers which influence the life principle, change the well-being of animal life. [165] This is effected by mechanical action upon their smallest particles by means of rubbing and shaking and through the addition of an indifferent substance, dry of fluid, are separated from each other. This process is called dynamizing, potentizing (development of medicinal power) and the products are dynamizations [166] or potencies in different degrees.

§ 270 Fifth Edition

Thus two drops of the fresh vegetable juice mingled with equal parts of alcohol are diluted with ninety-eight drops of alcohol and potentized by means of two succussions, whereby the first development of power is formed and this process is repeated through twenty-nine more phials, each of which is filled three-quarters full with ninety-nine drops of alcohol, and each succeeding phial is to be provided with one drop from the preceding phial (which has already been shaken twice) and is in its turn twice shaken, [267] and in the same manner at last the thirtieth development of power (potentized decillionth dilution X) which is the one most generally used.

§ 270 Sixth Edition

In order to best obtain this development of power, a small part of the substance to be dynamized, say one grain, is triturated for three hours with three times one hundred grains sugar of milk according to the method described below [168] up to the one-millionth part in powder form. For reasons given below (b) one grain of this powder is dissolved in 500 drops of a mixture of one part of alcohol and four parts of distilled water, of which one drop is put in a vial. To this are added 100 drops of pure alcohol [169] and given one hundred strong succussions with the hand against a hard but elastic body. [170] This is the medicine in the first degree of dynamization with which small sugar globules [171] may then be moistened [172] and quickly spread on blotting paper to dry and kept in a well-corked vial with the sign of (I) degree of potency. Only one [173] globule of this is taken for further dynamization, put in a second new vial (with a drop a water in order to dissolve it) and then with 100 powerful successions.

With this alcoholic medicinal fluid globules are again moistened, spread upon blotting paper and dried quickly, put into a well-stoppered vial and protected from heat and sun light and given the sign (II) of the second potency. And in this way the process is continued until the twenty-ninth is reached. Then with 100 drops of alcohol by means of 100 successions, an alcoholic medicinal fluid is formed with which the thirtieth dynamization degree is given to properly moistened and dried sugar globules.

By means of this manipulation of crude drugs are produced preparations which only in this way reach the full capacity to forcibly influence the suffering parts of the sick organism. In this way, by means of similar artificial morbid affection, the influence of the natural disease on the life principle present within is neutralized. By means of this mechanical procedure, provided it is carried out regularly according to the above teaching, a change is effected in the given drug, which in its crude state shows itself only as material, at times as unmedicinal material but by means of such higher and higher dynamization, it is changed and subtlized at last into spirit-like [174] medicinal power, which, indeed, in itself does not fall within our senses but for which the medicinally prepared globule, dry, but more so when dissolved in water, becomes the carrier, and in this condition, manifests the healing power of this invisible force in the sick body.

§ 271 Fifth Edition

All other substances adapted for medicinal use – except sulphur, which has of late years been only employed in the form of a highly diluted (X) tincture – as pure or oxidized and sulphuretted metals and other minerals, petroleum, phosphorus, as also parts and juices of plants that can only be obtained in the dry state, animal substances, neutral salts, etc., all these are first to be potentized by trituration for three hours, up to the millionfold pulverulent attenuation, and of this one grain is to be dissolved, and brought to the thirtieth development of power through twenty-seven attenuating phials, in the same manner as the vegetable juices. [175]

§ 271 Sixth Edition

If the physician prepares his homoeopathic medicines himself, as he should reasonably do in order to save men from sickness, [176] he may use the fresh plant itself, as but little of the crude article is required, if he does not need the expressed juice perhaps for purposes of healing. He takes a few grains in a mortar and with 100 grains sugar of milk three distinct times brings them to the one-millionth trituration (§ 270) before further potentizing of a small portion of this by means of shaking is undertaken, a procedure to be observed also with the rest of crude drugs of either dry or oily nature.

§ 272 Fifth Edition

In no case is it requisite to administer more than one single, simple medicinal substance at one time. [177]

§ 272 Sixth Edition

Such a globule, [178] placed dry upon the tongue, is one of the smallest doses for a moderate recent case of illness. Here but few nerves are touched by the medicine. A similar globule, crushed with some sugar of milk and dissolved in a good deal of water (§ 247) and stirred well before every administration will produce a far more powerful medicine for the use of several days. Every dose, no matter how minute, touches, on the contrary, many nerves.

§ 273 Fifth Edition

It is not conceivable how the slightest dubiety could exist as to whether it was more consistent with nature and more rational to prescribe a single well-known medicine at one time in a disease, or a mixture of several differently acting drugs.

§ 273 Sixth Edition

In no case under treatment is it necessary and therefore not permissible to administer to a patient more than one single, simple medicinal substance at one time. It is inconceivable how the slightest doubt could exist as to whether it was more consistent with nature and more rational to prescribe a single, simple [179] medicine at one time in a disease or a mixture of several differently acting drugs. It is absolutely not allowed in homoeopathy, the one true, simple and natural art of healing, to give the patient at one time two different medicinal substance.

§ 274

As the true physician finds in simple medicines, administered singly and uncombined, all that he can possibly desire (artificial disease-force which are able by homoeopathic power completely to overpower, extinguish, and permanently cure natural diseases), he will, mindful of the wise maxim that "it is wrong to attempt to employ complex means when simple means suffice," never think of giving as a remedy any but a single, simple medicinal substance; for these reasons also, because even though the simple medicines were thoroughly proved with respect to their pure peculiar effects on the unimpaired healthy state of man, it is yet impossible to foresee how two and more medicinal substances might, when compounded, hinder and alter each other's actions on the human body; and because, on the other hand, a simple medicinal substance when used in diseases, the totality of whose symptoms is accurately known, renders efficient aid by itself alone, if it be homoeopathically selected; and supposing the worst case to happen, that it was not chosen in strict conformity to similarity of symptoms, and therefore does no good, it is yet so far useful that it promoted our knowledge of therapeutic agents, because, by the new symptoms excited by it in such a case, those symptoms which this medicinal substance had already shown in experiments on the healthy human body are confirmed, an advantage that is lost by the employment of all compound remedies. [180]

§ 275

The suitableness of a medicine for any given case of disease does not depend on its accurate homoeopathic selection alone, but likewise on the proper size, or rather smallness, of the dose. If we give too strong a dose of a medicine which may have been even quite homoeopathically chosen for the morbid state before us, it must, notwithstanding the inherent beneficial character of its nature, prove injurious by its mere magnitude, and by the unnecessary, too strong impression which, by virtue of its homoeopathic similarity of action, it makes upon the vital force which it attacks and, through the vital force, upon those parts of the organism which are the most sensitive, and are already most affected by the natural disease.

§ 276 Fifth Edition

For this reason, a medicine, even though it may be homoeopathically suited to the case of disease, does harm in every dose that is too large, the more harm the larger the dose, and by the magnitude of the dose it does more harm the greater its homoeopathicity and the higher the potency [181] selected, and it does much more injury than any equally large dose of a medicine that is unhomoeopathic, and in no respect adapted (allopathic) to the morbid state; for in the former case the so-called homoeopathic aggravation (§§157-160) – that is to say, the very analogous medicinal disease produced by the vital force stirred up by the excessively large dose of medicine, in the parts of the organism that are most suffering and most irritated by the original disease – which medicinal disease, had it been of appropriate intensity, would have gently effected a cure – rises to an injurious height; [182] the patient, to be sure, no longer suffers from the original disease, for that has been homoeopathically eradicated, but he suffers all the more from the excessive medicinal disease and from useless exhaustion of his strength.

§ 276 Sixth Edition

For this reason, a medicine, even though it may be homoeopathically suited to the case of disease, does harm in every dose that is too large, the more harm the larger the dose, and by the magnitude of the dose and in strong doses' it does more harm the greater its homoeopathicity and the higher the potency1 selected, and it does much more injury than any equally large dose of a medicine that is unhomoeopathic, and in no respect adapted to the morbid state (allopathic).

Too large doses of an accurately chosen homoeopathic medicine, and especially when frequently repeated, bring about much trouble as a rule. They put the patient not seldom in danger of life or make this disease almost incurable. They do indeed extinguish the natural disease so far as the sensation of the life principle is concerned and the patient no longer suffers from the original disease from the moment the too strong dose of the homoeopathic medicine acted upon him but he is in consequence more ill with the similar but more violent medicinal disease which is most difficult to destroy.2

1 The praise bestowed of late years by some homoeopathists on the larger doses is owing to this, either that they chose low dynamizations of the medicine to be administered (as I myself used to do twenty years ago, from nor knowing any better), or that the medicines selected were not homoeopathic and imperfectly prepared by their manufacturers.

2 Thus, the continuous use of aggressive allopathic large doses of mercurials against syphilis develops almost incurable maladies, when yet one or several doses of a mild but active mercurial preparation would certainly have radically cured in a few days the whole venereal disease, together with the chancre, provided it had not been destroyed by external measures (as is always done by allopathy). In the same way, the allopath gives Peruvian bark and quinine in intermittent fever daily in very large doses, where they are correctly indicated and where one very small dose of a highly potentized China would unfailingly help (in marsh intermittents and even in persons who were not affected by any evi-

dent psoric disease). A chronic China malady (coupled at the same time with the development of psora) is produced, which, if it dose not gradually kill the patient by damaging the internal important vital organs, especially spleen and liver, will put him, nevertheless suffering for years in a sad state of health. A homoeopathic antidote for such a misfortune produced by abuse of large doses of homoeopathic remedies is hardly conceivable.

§ 277
For the same reason, and because a medicine, provided the dose of it was sufficiently small, is all the more salutary and almost marvellously efficacious the more accurately homoeopathic its selection has been, a medicine whose selection has been accurately homoeopathic must be all the more salutary the more its dose is reduced to the degree of minuteness appropriate for a gentle remedial effect.

§ 278 Fifth Edition
Here the question arises, what is this most suitable degree of minuteness for sure and gentle remedial effect; how small, in other words, must be the dose of each individual medicine, homoeopathically selected for a case of disease, to effect the best cure? To solve this problem, and to determine for every particular medicine, what dose of it will suffice for homoeopathic therapeutic purposes and yet be so minute that the gentlest and most rapid cure may be thereby obtained – to solve this problem is, as may easily be conceived, not the work off theoretical speculation; not by fine-spun reasoning, not by specious sophistry can we expect to obtain the solution of this problem. Pure experiment, careful observation, and accurate experience can alone determine this; and it were absurd to adduce the large doses of unsuitable (allopathic) medicines of the old system, which do not touch the diseased side of the organism homoeopathically, but only attack the parts unaffected by the disease, in opposition to what pure experience pronounces respecting the smallness of the doses required for homoeopathic cures.

§ 278 Sixth Edition
Here the question arises, what is this most suitable degree of minuteness for sure and gentle remedial effect; how small, in other words, must be the dose of each individual medicine, homoeopathically selected for a case of disease, to effect the best cure? To solve this problem, and to determine for every particular medicine, what dose of it will suffice for homoeopathic therapeutic purposes and yet be so minute that the gentlest and most rapid cure may be thereby obtained – to solve this problem is, as may easily be conceived, not the work off theoretical speculation; not by fine-spun reasoning, not by specious sophistry can we expect to obtain the solution of this problem. It is just as impossible as to tabulate in advance all imaginable cases. Pure experiment, careful observation of the sensitiveness of each patient, and accurate experience can alone determine this; and it were absurd to adduce the large doses of unsuitable (allopathic) medicines of the old system, which do not touch the diseased side of the organism homoeopathically, but only attack the parts unaffected by the disease, in opposition to what pure experience pronounces respecting the smallness of the doses required for homoeopathic cures.

§ 279 Fifth Edition

This pure experience shows UNIVERSALLY, that if the disease do not manifestly depend on a considerable deterioration of an important viscus (even though it belong to the chronic and complicated diseases), and if during the treatment all other alien medicinal influences are kept away from the patients, the dose of the homoeopathically selected remedy can never be prepared so small that it shall not be stronger than the natural disease, and shall not be able to overpower, extinguish and cure it, at least in part as long as it is capable of causing some, though but a slight preponderance of its own symptoms over those of the disease resembling it (slight homoeopathic aggravation, (§§ 157-160) immediately after its ingestion.

§ 279 Sixth Edition
This pure experience shows UNIVERSALLY, that if the disease do not manifestly depend on a considerable deterioration of an important viscus (even though it belong to the chronic and complicated diseases), and if during the treatment all other alien medicinal influences are kept away from the patients, the dose of the homoeopathically selected and highly potentized remedy for the beginning of treatment of an important, especially chronic disease can never be prepared so small that it shall not be stronger than the natural disease and shall not be able to overpower it, at least in part and extinguish it from the sensation of the principle of life and thus make a beginning of a cure.

§ 280 Fifth Edition
This incontrovertible axiom of experience is the standard of measurement by which the doses of all homoeopathic medicines, without exception, are to be reduced to such an extent that after their ingestion, they shall excite a scarcely observable homoeopathic aggravation, let the diminution of the dose go ever so far, and appear ever so incredible to the materialistic ideas of ordinary physicians; [183] their idle declamations must before the verdict of unerring experience.

§ 280 Sixth Edition
The dose of the medicine that continues serviceable without producing new troublesome symptoms is to be continued while gradually ascending, so long as the patient with general improvement, begins to feel in a mild degree the return of one or several old original complaints. This indicates an approaching cure through a gradual ascending of the moderate doses modified each time by succussion (§ 247). It indicates that the vital principal no longer needs to be affected by the similar medicinal disease in order to lose the sensation of the natural disease (§ 148). It indicates that the life principle now free from the natural disease begins to suffer only something of the medicinal disease hitherto known as homoeopathic aggravation.

§ 281 Fifth Edition
Every patient is, especially in his diseased point, capable of being influenced in an incredible degree by medicinal agents corresponding by similarity of action; and there is no person, be he ever so robust, and even though he be affected only with a chronic or so-called local disease, who will not soon experience the desired change in the affected part, if he take the salutary, homoeopathically suited medicine in the smallest conceivable dose, who, in a word, will not thereby be much more altered in his health than a healthy infant of but a day old would be.

How insignificant and ridiculous is mere theoretical scepticism in opposition to this unerring, infallible experimental proof!

§ 281 Sixth Edition
In order to be convinced of this, the patient is left without any medicine for eight, ten of fifteen days, meanwhile giving him only some powders of sugar of milk. If the few last complaints are due to the medicine simulating the former original disease symptoms, then these complaints will disappear in a few days or hours. If during these days without medicine, while continuing good hygienic regulations nothing more of the original disease is seen, he is probably cured. But if in the later days traces of the former morbid symptoms should show themselves, they are remnants of the original disease not wholly extinguished, which must be treated with renewed higher potencies of the remedy as directed before. If a cure is to follow, the first small doses must likewise be again gradually raised higher, but less and more slowly in patients where considerable irritability is evident than in those of less susceptibility, where the advance to higher dosage may be more rapid. There are patients whose impressionability compared to that of the insusceptible ones is like the ratio as 1000 to 1.

§ 282 Fifth Edition
The smallest possible dose of homoeopathic medicine capable of producing only the very slightest homoeopathic aggravation, will, because it has the power of exciting symptoms bearing the greatest possible resemblance to the original disease (but yet stronger even in the minute dose), attack principally and almost solely the parts in the organism that are already affected, highly irritated, and rendered excessively susceptible to such a similar stimulus, and will alter the vital force that rules in them to a state of very similar artificial disease, somewhat greater in degree than the natural one was; this artificial disease will substitute itself for the natural (the original) disease, so that the living organism now suffers from the artificial medicinal disease alone, which, from its nature and owing to the minuteness of the dose, will soon be extinguished by the vital force that is striving to return to the normal state, and (if the disease were only an acute one) the body is left perfectly free from disease – that is to say, quite well.

§ 282 Sixth Edition
It would be a certain sign that the doses were altogether too large, if during treatment, especially in chronic disease, the first dose should bring forth a so-called homoeopathic aggravation, that is, a marked increase of the original morbid symptoms first discovered and in the same way every repeated dose (§ 247) however modified somewhat by shaking before its administration (i.e., more highly dynamized). [184]

§ 283 Fifth Edition
Now, in order to act really in conformity with nature, the true physician will prescribe his well-selected homoeopathic medicine only in exactly as small a dose as will just suffice to over power and annihilate the disease before him – in a dose of such minuteness, that if human fallibility should betray him into administering an inappropriate medicine, the injury, accruing from its nature being unsuited to the disease will be diminished to a mere trifle; moreover the harm done by the smallest possible dose is so slight, that it may be immediately extinguished and

repaired by the natural vital powers, and by the speedy administration of a remedy more suitable selected according to similarity of action, and given also in the smallest dose.

§ 283 Sixth Edition

In order to work wholly according to nature, the true healing artist will prescribe the accurately chosen homoeopathic medicine most suitable in all respects in so small a dose on account of this alone. For should he be misled by human weakness to employ an unsuitable medicine, the disadvantage of its wrong relation to the disease would be so small that the patient could through his own vital powers and by means of early opposition (§ 249) of the correctly chosen remedy according to symptom similarly (and this also in the smallest dose) rapidly extinguish and repair it.

§ 284 Fifth Edition

The action of a dose, moreover, dose not diminish in the direct ratio of the quantity of material medicine contained in the dilutions used in homoeopathic practice. Eight drops of the tincture of a medicine to the dose do not produce four times as much effect on the human body as two drops, but only about twice the effect that is produced by two drops to the dose. In like manner, one drop of a mixture of a drop of the tincture with ten drops of some unmedicinal fluid, when taken, will not produce ten times more effect than one drop of mixture ten times more attenuated, but only about (scarcely) twice as strong an effect, and so on, in the same ratio – so that a drop of the lowest dilution must, and really does, display still a very considerable action. [185]

§ 284 Sixth Edition

Besides the tongue, mouth and stomach, which are most commonly affected by the administration of medicine, the nose and respiratory organs are receptive of the action of medicines in fluid form by means of olfaction and inhalation through the mouth. But the whole remaining skin of the body clothed with epidermis, is adapted to the action of medicinal solutions, especially if the inunction is connected with simultaneous internal administration. [186]

§ 285 Fifth Edition

The diminution of the dose essential for homoeopathic use, will also be promoted by diminishing its volume, so that, if, instead of a drop of a medicinal dilution, we take but quite a small part [187] of such a drop for a dose, the object of diminishing the effect still further will be very effectually attained; and that this will be the case may be readily conceived for this reason, because with the smaller volume of the dose but few nerves of the living organism can be touched, whereby the power of the medicine is certainly also communicated to the whole organism, but it is a weaker power.

§ 285 Sixth Edition

In this way, the cure of very old disease may be furthered by the physician applying externally, rubbing it in the back, arms, extremities, the same medicine he gives internally and which showed itself curatively. In doing so, he must avoid parts subject to pain or spasm or skin eruption. [188]

§ 286 Fifth Edition

For the same reason the effect of a homoeopathic dose of medicine increases, the greater the quantity of fluid in which it is dissolved when administered to the patient, although the actual amount of medicine it contains remains the same. For in this case, when the medicine is taken, it comes in contact with a much larger surface of sensitive nerves responsive to the medicinal action. Although theorists may imagine there should be a weakening of the action of dose of medicine by its dilution with a large quantity of liquid, experience asserts exactly the opposite, at all events when the medicines are employed homoeopathically. [189]

§ 286 Sixth Edition

The dynamic force of minerals magnets, electricity and galvanism act no less powerfully upon our life principle and they are not less homoeopathic than the properly so-called medicines which neutralize disease by taking them through the mouth, or by rubbing them on the skin or by olfaction. There may be diseases, especially diseases of sensibility and irritability, abnormal sensations, and involuntary muscular movements which may be cured by those means. But the more certain way of applying the last two as well as that of the so-called electromagnetic lies still very much in the dark to make homoeopathic use of them. So far both electricity and Galvanism have been used only for palliation to the great damage of the sick. The positive, pure action of both upon the healthy human body have until the present time been but little tested.

§ 287 Fifth Edition

But in this increase of action by the mixture of the dose of medicine with a larger quantity of liquid (before its ingestion), the result is vastly different whether the mixture of the dose of medicine with a certain quantity of liquid is performed merely superficially and imperfectly, or so uniformly and intimately [190] that the smallest portion of the diluting fluid received the same quantity of medicine in proportion as all the rest; for the latter becomes much more medicinally powerful by the diluting mixture than the former. From this every one will be able to judge for himself how to proceed with the regulation of the homoeopathic medicinal doses when he desires to diminish their medicinal action as much as possible, in order to make them suitable for the most sensitive patients. [191]

§ 287 Sixth Edition

The powers of the magnet for healing purposes can be employed with more certainty according to the positive effects detailed in the Materia Medica Pura under north and south pole of a powerful magnetic bar. Though both poles are alike powerful, they nevertheless oppose each other in the manner of their respective action. The doses may be modified by the length of time of contact with one or the other pole, according as the symptoms of either north or south pole are indicated. As antidote to a too violent action the application of a plate of polished zinc will suffice.

§ 288 Fifth Edition

The action of medicines in the liquid from [192] upon the living human body takes place in such a penetrating manner, spreads out from the point of the sensitive fibers provided with nerves whereto the medicine is first applied with such inconceivable rapidity and so universally through all parts of the living body, that this action of the medicine must be denominated a spirit-like (a dynamic, virtual) action.

§ 288 Sixth Edition

I find it yet necessary to allude here to animal magnetism, as it is termed, or rather Mesmerism (as it should be called in deference to Mesmer, its first founder) which differs so much in its nature from all other therapeutic agents. This curative force, often so stupidly denied and disdained for a century, acts in different ways. It is a marvellous, priceless gift of God to mankind by means of which the strong will of a well intentioned person upon a sick one by contact and even without this and even at some distance, can bring the vital energy of the healthy mesmerizer endowed with this power into another person dynamically (just as one of the poles of a powerful magnetic rod upon a bar of steel).

It acts in part by replacing in the sick whose vital force within the organism is deficient here and there, in part also in other parts where the vital force has accumulated too much and keeps up irritating nervous disorders it turns it aside, diminishes and distributes it equally and in general extinguishes the morbid condition of the life principle of the patient and substitutes in its place the normal of the mesmerist acting powerfully upon him, for instance, old ulcers, amaurosis, paralysis of single organs and so forth. Many rapid apparent cures performed in all ages, by mesmerizers endowed with great natural power, belong to this class. The effect of communicated human power upon the whole human organism was most brilliantly shown, in the resuscitation of persons who had lain some time apparently dead, by the most powerful sympathetic will of a man in full vigor of vital energy, [193] and of this kind of resurrection history records many undeniable examples.

If the mesmerizing person of either sex capable at the same time of a good-natured enthusiasm (even its degeneration into bigotry, fanaticism, mysticism or philanthropic dreaming) will be empowered all the more with this philanthropic self-sacrificing performance to direct exclusively the power of his commanding good will to the recipient requiring his help and at the same time to concentrate these, he may at times perform apparent miracles.

§ 289 Fifth Edition
Every part of our body that possesses the sense of touch is also capable of receiving the influences, and of propagating their power to all other parts. [194]

§ 289 Sixth Edition
All the above-mentioned methods of practicing mesmerism depend upon influx of more or less vital force into the patient, and hence are termed positive mesmerism. [195] An opposite mode of employing mesmerism, however, as it produces just the contrary effect, deserves to be termed negative mesmerism. To this belong the passes which are used to rouse from the somnambulic sleep, as also all the manual processes known by the names of soothing and ventilating. This discharge by means of negative mesmerism of the vital force accumulated to excess in individual parts of the system of undebilitated persons is most surely and simply performed by making a very rapid motion or the flat extended hand, held parallel to, and about an inch distant from the body, from the top of the head to the tips of the toes. [196] The more rapidly this pass is made, so much the more effectually will the discharge be effected. Thus, for instance, in the case where a previously healthy woman, [197] from the sudden suppression of her catamenia by a violent mental shock, lies to all appearance dead, the vital force which is probably accumulated in the precordial region, will, by such a rapid

negative pass, be discharged and its equilibrium throughout the whole organism restored. So that the resuscitation generally follows, immediately. [198] In like manner, a gentle, less rapid, negative pass diminishes the excessive restlessness and sleeplessness accompanied with anxiety sometimes produced in very irritable persons by a too powerful positive pass, etc.

§ 290 Fifth Edition*
Besides the stomach, the tongue and the mouth are the parts most susceptible to the medicinal influences; but the interior of the nose is more especially so, and the rectum, the genitals, as also all particularly sensitive parts of our body are almost equally capable of receiving the medicinal action; hence also, parts that are destitute of skin, wounded or ulcerated spots permit the powers of medicines to exercise almost as penetrating an action upon the organism as if the medicine had been taken by the mouth or still better by olfaction and inhalation.

* § 290 corresponds to some extent to § 284 of the Sixth Edition.

§ 290 Sixth Edition
Here belongs also the so-called massage of vigorous good-natured person given to a chronic invalid, who, though cured, still suffers from loss of flesh, weakness of digestion and lack of sleep due to slow convalescence. The muscles of the limbs, breast and back, separately grasped and moderately pressed and kneaded arouse the life principle to reach and restore the tone of the muscles and blood and lymph vessels. The mesmeric influences of this procedure is the chief feature and it must not be used to excess in patients still hypersensitive.

§ 291 Fifth Edition
Even those organs which have lost their peculiar sense, e.g., a tongue and palate that have lost the faculty of tasting, or a nose that has lost the faculty of smelling, communicate the power of the medicine that acts first on them alone not less perfectly to all the other organs of the body.

§ 291 Sixth Edition
Baths of pure water prove themselves partly palliative, partly as homoeopathic serviceable aids in restoring health in acute diseases as well as in convalescence of cured chronic patients with proper consideration of the conditions of the convalescent and the temperature of the bath, its duration and repetition. But even if well applied, they may bring only physically beneficial changes in the sick body, in themselves they are no true medicine. The lukewarm baths at 25 to 27? serve to arouse the slumbering sensibility of fibre in the apparent dead (frozen, drowned, suffocated) which benumbed the sensation of the nerves. Though only palliative, still they often prove themselves sufficiently active, especially when given in conjunction with coffee and rubbing with the hands. They may give homoeopathic aid in cases where the irritability is very unevenly distributed and accumulated too unevenly in some organs as is the case in certain hysteric spasms and infantile convulsions. In the same way, cold baths 10 to 6? in persons cured medically of chronic diseases and with deficiency of vital heat, act as an homoeopathic aid. By instantaneous and later with repeated immersions they act as a palliative restorative of the tone of the exhausted fibre. For this purpose, such baths are to be used for more than momentary duration, rather for minutes and of gradually lowered temperature, they are a palliative, which, since it acts

only physically has no connection with the disadvantage of a reverse action to be feared afterwards, as takes place with dynamic medicinal palliatives.

§ 292 Fifth Edition
Even the external surface of the body, covered as it is with skin and epidermis, is not insusceptible of the powers of medicines, especially those in a liquid form, but the most sensitive parts are also the most susceptible. [199]

§ 293 Fifth Edition
I find it necessary to allude here to animal magnetism, as it is termed, or rather mesmerism (as it should be called, out of gratitude to Mesmer, its first founder), which differs so much in its nature from all other therapeutic agents. This curative power, often so stupidly denied, which streams upon a patient by the contact of a well-intentioned person powerfully exerting his will, either acts homoeopathically, by the production of symptoms similar to those of the diseased state to be cured; and for this purpose a single pass made, without much exertion of the will, with the palms of the hands not too slowly from the top of the head downwards over the body to the tips of the toes, [200] is serviceable in, for instance, uterine haemorrhages, even in the last stage when death seems approaching; or it is useful by distributing the vital force uniformly throughout the organism, when it is in abnormal excess in one part and deficient in other parts, for example, in rush of blood to the head and sleepless, anxious restlessness of weakly persons, etc., by means of a similar, single, but somewhat stronger pass; or for the immediate communication and restoration of the vital force to some one weakened part or to the whole organism, – an object that cannot be attained so certainly and with so little interference with the other medicinal treatment by any other agent besides mesmerism. If it is wished to supply a particular part with the vital force, this is effected by concentrating a very powerful and well-intentioned will for the purpose, and placing the hands or tips of the fingers on the chronically weakened parts, whither an internal chronic dyscrasia has transferred its important local symptom, as, for example, in the case of old ulcers, amaurosis, paralysis of certain limbs, etc. [201] Many rapid apparent cures performed in all ages, by mesmerizers endowed with great natural power, belong to this class. The effect of communicated human power upon the whole human organism was most brilliantly shown, in the resuscitation of persons who had lain some time apparently dead, by the most powerful sympathetic will of a man in full vigor of vital force, [202] and of this kind of resurrection history records many undeniable examples.

§ 294 Fifth Edition*
All the above-mentioned methods of practicing mesmerism depend upon an influx of more or less vital force into the patient, and hence are termed positive mesmerism. [203] An opposite mode of employing mesmerism, however, as it produces just the contrary effect, deserves to be termed negative mesmerism. To this belong the passes which are used to rouse from the somnambulic sleep, as also all the manual processes known by the names of soothing and ventilating. This discharge by means of negative mesmerism of the vital force accumulated to excess in individual parts of the system of undebiliated persons is most surely and simply performed by making a very rapid motion of the flat extended hand, held parallel to, and about an inch distant from the body, from the top of the

head to the tips of the toes. [204] The more rapidly this pass is made, so much the more effectually will the discharge be effected. Thus, for instance, in the case where a previously healthy woman, [205] from the sudden suppression of her catamenia by a violent mental shock, lies to all appearance dead, the vital force which is probably accumulated in the precordial region, will by such a rapid negative pass, be discharged and its equilibrium throughout the whole organism restored, so that the resuscitation generally follows immediately. [206] In like manner, a gentle, less rapid, negative pass diminishes the excessive restlessness and sleeplessness accompanied with anxiety sometimes produced in very irritable persons by a too powerful positive pass, etc.

* This Section corresponds to § 289 of the Sixth Edition.

Notes

[1] I know not, therefore, how it was possible for physicians at the sick-bed to allow themselves to suppose that, without most carefully attending to the symptoms and being guided by them in the treatment, they ought to seek and could discover, only in the hidden and unknown interior, what there was to be cured in the disease, arrogantly and ludicrously pretending that they could, without paying much attention to the symptoms, discover the alteration that had occurred in the invisible interior, and set it to rights with (unknown!) medicines, and that such a procedure as this could alone be called radical and rational treatment.

Is not, then, that which is cognizable by the senses in diseases through the phenomena it displays, the disease itself in the eyes of the physician, since he never can see the spiritual being that produces the disease, the vital force? nor is it necessary that he should see it, but only that he should ascertain its morbid actions, in order that he may thereby be enabled to cure the disease. What else will the old school search for in the hidden interior of the organism, as a prima causa morbi, whilst they reject as an object of cure and contemptuously despise the sensible and manifest representation of the disease, the symptoms, that so plainly address themselves to us? What else do they wish to cure in disease but these?*

* The physician whose researches are directed towards the hidden relations in the interior of the organism, may daily err; but the homoeopathist who grasps with requisite carefulness the whole group of symptoms, possesses a sure guide; and if he succeed in removing the whole group of symptoms he has likewise most assuredly destroyed the internal, hidden cause of the disease.

[2] It is not necessary to say that every intelligent physician would first remove this where it exists; the indisposition thereupon generally ceases spontaneously. He will remove from the room strong-smelling flowers, which have a tendency to cause syncope and hysterical sufferings; extract from the cornea the foreign body that excites inflammation of the eye; loosen the over-tight bandage on a wounded limb that threatens to cause mortification, and apply a more suitable one; lay bare and put ligature on the wounded artery that produces fainting; endeavour to promote the expulsion by vomiting of belladonna berries etc., that may have been swallowed; extract foreign substances that may have got into the orifices of the body (the nose, gullet, ears, urethra, rectum, vagina); crush the vesical calculus; open the imperforate anus of the newborn infant, etc.

[3] In all times, the old school physicians, not knowing how else to give relief, have sought to combat and if possible to suppress by medicines, here and there, a single symptom from among a number in diseases – a one-sided procedure, which, under the name of symptomatic treatment, has justly excited universal contempt, because by it, not only was nothing gained, but much harm was inflicted. A single one of the symptoms present is no more the disease itself than a foot is the man himself. This procedure was so much the more reprehensible, that such a single symptom was only treated by an antagonistic remedy (therefore only in an enantiopathic and palliative manner), whereby, after a slight alleviation, it was subsequently only rendered all the worse.

[4] When a patient has been cured of his disease by a true physician, in such a manner that no trace of the disease, no morbid symptom, remains, and all the signs of health have permanently returned, how can anyone, without offering an insult to common sense, affirm in such an individual the whole bodily disease still remains interior? And yet the chief of the old school, Hufeland, asserts this in the following words: "Homoeopathy can remove symptoms, but the disease remains." (Vide Homoopathie, p.27, 1, 19.) This he maintains partly from mortification at the progress made by homoeopathy to the benefits of mankind, partly because he still holds thoroughly material notions respecting disease, which he is still unable to regard as a state of being of the organism wherein it is dynamically altered by the morbidly deranged vital force, as an altered state of health, but he views the disease as a something material, which after the cure is completed, may still remain lurking in some corner in the interior of the body, in order, some day during the most vigorous health, to burst forth at its pleasure with its material presence! So dreadful is still the blindness of the old pathology! No wonder that it could only produce a system of therapeutics which is solely occupied with scouring out the poor patient.

[5] It is dead, and only subject to the power of the external physical world; it decays, and is again resolved into its chemical constituents.

[6] Materia peccans!

[7] What is dynamic influence, – dynamic power? Our earth, by virtue of a hidden invisible energy, carries the moon around her in twenty-eight days and several hours, and the moon alternately, in definite fixed hours (deducting certain differences which occur with the full and new moon) raises our northern seas to flood tide and again correspondingly lowers them to ebb. Apparently this takes place not through material agencies, not through mechanical contrivances, as are used for products of human labor; and so we see numerous other events about us as results of the action of one substance on another substance without being able to recognize a sensible connection between cause and effect. Only the cultured, practised in comparison and deduction, can form for himself a kind of supra-sensual idea sufficient to keep all that is material or mechanical in his thoughts from such concepts. He calls such effects dynamic, virtual, that is, such as result from absolute, specific, pure energy and action of he one substance upon the other substance.

For instance, the dynamic effect of the sick-making influences upon healthy man, as well as the dynamic energy of the medicines upon the principle of life in the restoration of health is nothing else than infection and so not in any way material, not in any way mechanical. Just as the energy of a magnet attracting a piece of iron or steel is not material, not mechanical. One sees that the piece of iron is attracted by one pole of the magnet, but how it is done is not seen. This invisible energy of the magnet does not require mechanical (material) auxiliary means, hook or lever, to attract the iron. The magnet draws to itself and this acts upon the piece of iron or upon a steel needle by means of a purely immaterial invisible, conceptual, inherent energy, that is, dynamically, and communicates to the steel needle the magnetic energy equally invisibly (dynamically). The steel needle becomes itself magnetic, even at a distance when the magnet does not touch it, and magnetises other steel needles with the same magnetic property (dynamically) with which it had been endowed previously by the magnetic rod, just as a child with small-pox or measles communicates to a near, untouched healthy child in an invisible manner (dynamically) the small-pox or measles, that is, infects it at a distance without anything material from the infective child going or capable of going to the one to be infected. A purely specific conceptual influence communicated to the near child small-pox or measles in the same way as the magnet communicated to the near needle the magnetic property.

In a similar way, the effect of medicines upon living man is to be judged. Substances, which are used as medicines, are medicines only in so far as they possess each its own specific energy to alter the well-being of man through dynamic, conceptual influence, by means of the living sensory fibre, upon the conceptual controlling principle of life. The medicinal property of those material substances which we call medicines proper, relates only to their energy to call out alterations in the well-being of animal life. Only upon this conceptual principle of life, depends their medicinal health-altering, conceptual (dynamic) influence. Just as the nearness of a magnetic pole can communicate only magnetic energy to the steel (namely, by a kind of infection) but cannot communicate other properties (for instance, more hardness or ductility, etc.). And thus every special medicinal substance alters through a kind of infection, that well-being of man in a peculiar manner exclusively its own and not in a manner peculiar to another medicine, as certainly as the nearness of the child ill with small-pox will communicate to a healthy child only small-pox and not measles. These medicines act upon our well-being wholly without communication of material parts of the medicinal substances, thus dynamically, as if through infection. Far more healing energy is expressed in a case in point by the smallest dose of the best dynamized medicines, in which there can be, according to calculation, only so little of material substance that its minuteness cannot be thought and conceived by the best arithmetical mind, than by large doses of the same medicine in substance. That smallest dose can therefore contain almost entirely only the pure, freely-developed, conceptual medicinal energy, and bring about only dynamically such great effects as can never be reached by the crude medicinal substances itself taken in large doses.

It is not in the corporal atoms of these highly dynamized medicines, nor their physical or mathematical surfaces (with which the higher energies of the dynamized medicines are being interpreted but vainly as still sufficiently material) that the medicinal energy is found. More likely, there lies invisible in the moistened globule or in its solution, an unveiled, liberated, specific, medicinal force contained in the medicinal substance which acts dynamically by contact with the living animal fibre upon the whole organism (without communicating to it anything material however highly attenuated) and acts more strongly the more free and more immaterial the energy has become through the dynamization.

Is it then so utterly impossible for our age celebrated for its wealth in clear thinkers to think of dynamic energy as something non-corporeal, since we see daily phenomena which cannot be explained in any other manner? If one looks upon something nauseous and becomes inclined to vomit, did a material emetic come into his stomach which compels him to this anti-peristaltic movement? Was it not solely the dynamic effect of the nauseating aspect upon his imagination? And if one raises his arm, does it occur *through a material visible instrument? a lever? Is it not solely the conceptual dynamic energy of his will which raises it?*

[8] How the vital force causes the organism to display morbid phenomena, that is, how it produces disease, it would be of no practical utility to the physician to know, and will forever remain concealed from him; only what it is necessary for him to know of the disease and what is fully sufficient for enabling him to cure it, has the Lord of life revealed to his senses.

[9] Most severe disease may be produced by sufficient disturbance of the vital force through the imagination and also cured by the same means.

[10] A warning dream, a superstitious fancy, or a solemn prediction that death would occur at a certain day or at a certain hour, has not unfrequently produced all the signs of commencing and increasing disease, of approaching death and death itself at the hour announced, which could not happen without the simultaneous production of the inward change (corresponding to the state observed internally); and hence in such cases all the morbid signs indicative of approaching death have frequently been dissipated by an identical cause, by some cunning deception or persuasion to a belief in the contrary, and health suddenly restored, which could not have happened without the removal, by means of this mortal remedy, of the internal and external morbid change that threatened death.

[11] It is only thus that God the preserver of mankind, could reveal His wisdom and goodness in reference to the cure of the disease to which man is liable here below, by showing to the physician what he had to remove in disease in order to annihilate them and thus re-establish health. But what would we think of His wisdom and goodness if He has shrouded in mysterious obscurity that which was to be cured in diseases (as is asserted by the dominant school of medicine, which affects to possess a supernatural insight into the nature of things), and shut it up in the hidden interior, and thus rendered it impossible for man to know the malady accurately, consequently impossible for him to cure it?

[12] The other possible mode of employing medicines for diseases besides these two is the allopathic method, in which medicines are given, whose symptoms have no direct pathological relation to the morbid state, neither similar nor opposite, but quite heterogeneous to the symptoms of the disease, is, as shown above, in the introduction (Review of the therapeutics, allopathy and palliative treatment that have hitherto been practiced in the old school of medicine), merely instinctive vital force, which, when made ill by noxious agents, strives to save itself at whatever sacrifice by the production and continuance of morbid irritation in the organism – an imitation, consequently, of the crude vital force which was implanted in our organism in order to preserve our life in health, in the most beautiful harmony; but when deranged by disease, was so constituted as to admit of being again changed to health (homoeopathically) by the intelligent physician, but not to cure itself, for which the little power it possesses is so far from being a pattern to be copied, that all the changes and symptoms it produces in the (morbidly deranged) organism are just the disease itself. But this injudicious system of therapeutics of the old school of medicine can no more be passed by unnoticed that can history omit to record the thousands of years of opposition to which mankind has been subjected under the irrational, despotic Governments.

[13] The other possible mode of employing medicines for diseases besides these two is the allopathic method, in which medicines are given, whose symptoms have no direct pathological relation to the morbid state, neither similar nor opposite, but quite heterogeneous to the symptoms of the disease. This procedure plays, as I have shown else-

where, an irresponsible murderous game with the life of the patient by means of dangerous, violent medicines, whose action is unknown and which are chosen on mere conjectures and given in large and frequent doses. Again, by means of painful operations, intended to lead the disease to other regions and taking the strength and vital juices of the patient, through evacuations above and below, sweat or salivation, but especially through squandering the irreplaceable blood, as is done by the reigning routine practice, used blindly and relentlessly, usually with the pretext that the physician should imitate and further the sick nature in its efforts to help itself, without considering how irrational it is, to imitate and further these very imperfect, mostly inappropriate efforts of the instinctive unintelligent vital energy which is implanted in our organism, so long as it is healthy to carry on life in harmonious development, but not to heal itself in disease. For, were it possessed of such a model ability, it would never have allowed the organism to get sick. When made ill by noxious agents, our life principle cannot do anything else than express its depression caused by disturbance of the regularity of its life, by symptoms, by means of which the intelligent physician is ask for aid. If this is not given, it strives to save by increasing the ailment, especially through violent evacuations, no matter what this entails, often with the largest sacrifices or destruction of life itself.

For the purpose of cure, the morbidly depressed vital energy possesses so little ability worthy of imitation since all changes and symptoms produced by it in the organism are the disease itself. What intelligent physician would want to imitate it with the intention to heal if he did not thereby sacrifice his patient?

[14] I do not mean that sort of experience of which the ordinary practitioners of the old school boast, after they have for years worked away with a lot of complex prescriptions on a number of diseases which they never carefully investigate, but which, faithful to their school, they consider as already described in works of systematic pathology, and dreamed that they could detect in them some imaginary morbific matter, or ascribe to them some other hypothetical internal abnormality. They always saw something in them, but knew not what it was they saw, and they got results, from the complex forces acting on an unknown object, that no human being but only a God could have unravelled – results from which nothing can be learned, no experience gained. Fifty years' experience of this sort is like fifty years of looking into a kaleidoscope filled with unknown colored objects, and perpetually turning round; thousands of ever changing figures and no accounting for them!

[15] Thus are cured both physical affections and moral maladies. How is it that in the early dawn the brilliant Jupiter vanishes from the gaze of the beholder? By a stronger very similar power acting on his optic nerve, the brightness of approaching day! – In situations replete with foetid odors, wherewith is it usual to soothe effectually the offended olfactory nerves? With snuff, that affects the sense of smell in a similar but stronger manner! No music, no sugared cake, which act on the nerves of other senses, can cure this olfactory disgust. How does the soldier cunningly stifle the piteous cries of him who runs the gauntlet from the ears of the compassionate bystanders? By the shrill notes of the fife commingled with the roll of the noisy drum! And the distant roar of the enemy's cannon that inspires his army with fear? By the loud boom of the big drum! For neither the one nor the other would the distribution of a brilliant piece of uniform nor a reprimand to the regiment suffice. In like manner, mourning and sorrow will be effaced from the mind by the account of another and still greater cause for sorrow happening to another, even though it be a mere fiction. The injurious consequences of too great joy will be removed by drinking coffee, which produces an excessive joyous state of mind.

Nations like the Germans, who have for centuries been gradually sinking deeper and deeper in soulless apathy and degrading serfdom, must first be trodden still deeper in the dust by the Western Conqueror, until their situation became intolerable; their mean opinion of themselves was thereby over-strained and removed; they again became alive to their dignity as men, and then, for the first time, they raised their heads as Germans.

[16] *The short duration of the action of the artificial morbific forces, which we term medicines, makes it possible that, although they are stronger than the natural diseases, they can yet be much more easily overcome by the vital force than can the weaker natural diseases, which solely in consequence of the longer, generally lifelong, duration of their action (psora, syphilis, sycosis), can never be vanquished and extinguished by it alone, until the physician affects the vital force in a stronger manner by an agent that produces a disease very similar, but stronger to wit a homoeopathic medicine, which, when taken (or smelt), is as it were, forced upon the unintelligent, instinctive vital force, and substituted in the place of the former natural morbid affection, by which means the vital force, and substituted in the place of the former natural morbid affection, by which means the vital force then remains merely medicinally ill, but only for a short time, because the action of the medicine (the time in which the medicinal disease excited by it run its course) does not last long. The cures of diseases of many years' duration (§ 46), by the occurrence of smallpox and measles (both of which run a course of only a few weeks), are processes of a similar character.*

[17] *The short duration of the action of the artificial morbific forces, which we term medicines, makes it possible that, although they are stronger than the natural diseases, they can yet be much more easily overcome by the vital force than can the weaker natural diseases, which solely in consequence of the longer, generally lifelong, duration of their action (psora, syphilis, sycosis), can never be vanquished and extinguished by it alone, until the physician affects the vital force in a stronger manner by an agent that produces a disease very similar, but stronger to wit a homoeopathic medicine. The cures of diseases of many years' duration (§ 46), by the occurrence of smallpox and measles (both of which run a course of only a few weeks), are processes of a similar character.*

[18] *When I call a disease a derangement of man's state of health, I am far from wishing thereby to give a hyperphysical explanation of the internal nature of disease generally, or of any case of disease in particular. It is only intended by this expression to intimate, what it can be proved diseases are not and cannot be, that they are not mechanical or chemical alterations of material substance of the body, and not dependant on a material morbific substance, but that they are merely spirit-like (conceptual) dynamic derangements of the life.*

[19] *A striking fact in corroboration of this is, that whilst previously to the year 1801, when the smooth scarlatina of Sydenham still occasionally prevailed epidemically among children, it attacked without exception all children who had escaped it in a former epidemic; in a similar epidemic which I witnessed in Konigslutter, on the contrary, all the children who took in time a very small dose of belladonna remained unaffected by this highly infectious infantile disease. If medicines can protect from a disease that is raging around, they must possess a vastly superior power of affecting our vital force.*

[20] *"Memoires et Observations," in the Description de l' Egpte, tom. i.*

[21] *But if treated with violent allopathic remedies, other diseases will be formed in its place which are more difficult and dangerous to life.*

[22] *Obs., lib. I, obs. 8.*

[23] *In Hufeland's Journal, xv, 2.*

[24] Chevalier, in Hufeland's Neuesten Annalen der franzosichen Heikunde, ii, p.192.
[25] Mania phthisi superveniens eam cum omnibus suis phaenomenis auffert, verum mox redit phthisis et occidit, abeunte mania. Reil Memorab., fasc. iii, v, p.171.
[26] In the Edinb. Med. Comment., pt. i, 1.
[27] John Hunter, On the veneral Disease, p.5.
[28] Rainey, in the Edinb. Med. Comment., iii, p.480.
[29] Very accurately described by Withering and Plenciz, but differing greatly from the purpura (or Roodvonk), which is often erroneously denominated scarlet fever. It is only of late year that the two, which were originally very different diseases, have come to resemble each other in their symptoms.
[30] Jenner, in Medicinische Annalen, August, 1800, p.747.
[31] In Hufeland's Journal der praktischen Arzneikunde, xx, 3, p.50.
[32] Loc. cit.
[33] Obs. phys. med., lib. ii, obs, 30.
[34] From careful experiments and cures of complex diseases of this kind, I am now firmly convinced that no real amalgamation of the two takes place, but that in such cases the one exists in the organism besides the other only, each in pairs that are adapted for it, and their cure will be completely effected by a judicious alternation of the best mercurial preparation, with the remedies specific for the psora, each given in the most suitable dose and form.
[35] Vide Transactions of a Society for the Improvement of Med. and Chir. Knowledge, ii.
[36] In Edinb. Med and Phys. Journ., 1805.
[37] In Med. and Phys. Journ., 1805.
[38] Opera, ii, p.i, cap. 10.
[39] In hufeland's Journal, xvii.
[40] For mercury, besides the morbid symptoms which by virtue of similarity can cure the venereal disease homoeopathically, has among its effects many others unlike those of syphilis, for instance, swelling and ulceration of bones, which, if it be employed in large doses, causes new maladies and commit great ravages in the body, especially when complicated with psora, as is so frequently the case.
[41] Vide, supra, § 26, note.
[42] Just as the image of a lamp's flame is rapidly overpowered and effaced from our retina by the stronger sunbeam impinging on the eye.
[43] Traite de l'inoculation, p.189.
[44] Heilkunde fur Mutter, p.384.
[45] Interpres clinicus, p.293.
[46] Neue Heilart der Kinderpocken. Ulm, 1769, p.68; and Specim., obs. No. 18.
[47] Op. cit.
[48] Nov. Act. Nat. cur., vol, I, obs. 22.
[49] Nachricht Von dem Krankeninstitut zu Erlangen, 1783.
[50] A new footnote is added here in the Sixth Edition, as follows:
This seems to be the reason for this beneficial remarkable fact namely that since the general distribution of Janner's Cow-pox vaccination, human small-pox never again appeared as epidemically or virulently as 40-45 years before when one city visited lost at least one-half and often three-quarters of its children by death of this miserable pestilence.
[51] Willian, Ueber die Kuhpockenimpfung, aus dem Engl., mit Zusatzen G.P. Muhry, Gottingen, 1808.

[52] Especially Clavier, Hurel and Desmormeaux, in the Bulletin des sciencs medicales, publie par les membres de l' Eure, 1808, also in the Journal de medicine continue, vol. xv, p.206.
[53] Balhorn, in Hufeland's Journal, 10, ii.
[54] Stevenson, in Duncan's Annals of Medicine, lustr. 2, vol. I, pt. 2, No. 9.
[55] In Hufeland's Journal, xxiii.
[56] On the Veneral Disease, p.4.
[57] Cullen's Elements of Practical Medicine, pt. 2, I, 3, ch. vii.
[58] Or at least that symptom was removed.
[59] In Hufeland's Journal, xx, 3, p.50.
[60] Rau, Ueber d. Werth des hom. Heidelb., 1824, p.85.
[61] And the exanthematous contagious principle present in the cow-pox lymph.
[62] Namely, small-pox and measles.
[63] Vide supra in the Introduction: A review of the Therapeutics, etc., and my book, Die Alloopathie, ein Wort der Warnung fur Kranke jeder Art, Leipzig, bei Baumgartner (translated in Hahnemann's Lesser Writings.)
[64] As if the establishment of a science, based only on observation of nature and pure experiment and experience idle speculation and scholastic vaporings could have a place.
[65] Up to the most recent times what is curable in sickness was supposed to be material that had to be removed since no one could conceive of a dynamic effect (§ 11 note) of morbific agencies, such as medicines exercise upon the life of the animal organism.
[66] To fill the measure of self infatuation to overflowing here were mixed (very learnedly) constantly more, indeed, many different medicines in so-called prescriptions to be administered in frequent and large doses and thereby the precious, easily-destroyed human life was endangered in the hands of these perverted ones. Especially so with seton, venesection, emetics, purgatives, plasters, fontanelles and cauterization.
[67] Review of the Therapeutics, etc.
[68] A fourth mode of employing medicines in diseases has been attempted to be created by means of Isopathy, as it is called – that is to say, a method of curing a given disease by the same contagious particle that produces it. But even granting this could be done, which would certainly be a valuable discovery, yet, after all, seeing that the virus is given to the patient highly potentized, and thereby, consequently, to a certain degree in an altered condition, the cure is effected only by opposing a simillimum to a simillimum.
[69] A third mode of employing medicines in diseases has been attempted to be created by means of Isopathy, as it is called – that is to say, a method of curing a given disease by the same contagious principle that produces it. But even granting this could be done, yet, after all, seeing that the virus is given to the patient highly potentized, and consequently, in an altered condition, the cure is effected only by opposing a simillimum to a simillimum.

To attempt to cure by means of the very same morbific potency (per Idem) contradicts all normal human understanding and hence all experience. Those who first brought Isopathy to notice, probably thought of the benefit which mankind received from cowpox vaccination by which the vaccinated individual is protected against future cowpox infection and as it were cured in advance. But both, cowpox and smallpox are only similar, in no way the same disease. In many respects they differ, namely in the more rapid course and mildness of cowpox and especially in this, that is never contagious to man by more nearness. Universal vaccination put an end to all epidemics of that deadly fearful smallpox to such an extent that the present generation does no longer possess a clear conception of the former frightful smallpox plague.

Moreover, in this way, undoubtedly, certain diseases peculiar to animals may give us remedies and thus happily enlarge our stock of homoeopathic remedies.

But to use a human morbific matter (a Psorin taken from the itch in man) as a remedy for the same itch or for evils arisen therefrom is –?

Nothing can result from this but trouble and aggravation of the disease.

[70] Little as physicians have hitherto been in the habit of observing accurately, the aggravation that so certainly follows such palliative treatment could not altogether escape their notice. A striking example of this is to be found in J. H. Schulze's Diss. qua corporis humani momentanearum alterationum specimina quoedam expenduntur, Hale, 1741, § 28. Willis bears testimony to something similar (Pharm. rat., § 7, cap. I, p.298): "Opiata dolores atroscissimos plerumque sedant atque indolentiam – procurant, camque – aliquamdiu et pro stato quodam tempore continuant, quo spatio elapso dolores mox recrusescunt et brevi ad sol itam ferociam augentur." And also at page 295: "Exactis opii viribus illico redeunt tormina, nec atrocitatem suam remittunt, nisi dum ab eodem pharmaco rursus incantuntur." In like manner J. Hunter (On the Venereal Disease, p.13) says that wine and cordials given to the weak increase the action without giving real strength, and the powers of the body are afterwards sunk proportionally as they have been raised, by which nothing can be gained, but a great deal may be lost.

[71] Vide Introduction.

[72] Vide Hufeland, in his pamphlet, Die Homoopathie, p.20.

[73] All usual palliatives given for the suffering of the sick have (as is seen here) as after-effects an increase of the same suffering and the older physicians had to repeat them in ever stronger doses in order to achieve a similar modification, which however, was never permanent and never sufficient to prevent an increased recurrence of the ailment. But Brousseau, who twenty-five years before contended against the senseless mixing of different drugs in prescription and thereby ending its reign in France, (for which mankind is grateful to him) introduced his so-called physiological system (without taking note of the homoeopathic method then already established), a method of treatment, while effectively lessening and permanently preventing the return of all the sufferings, was applicable to all diseases of mankind; a thing that the palliatives then in use were not capable of affecting.

Being able to heal disease with mild innocent remedies and thus establish health, Brousseau found the easier way to quiet the sufferings of patients more and more at the cost of their life and at last to extinguish life wholly – a method of treatment that, alas, seemed sufficient to his contemporaries. In the degree that the patient retains his strength will his ailments be apparent and the more intensely will he feel his pains. He moans and groans and cries out and calls for help more and more vociferously so that the physician cannot come any too soon to give relief. Brousseau needed only to depress the vital force, to lessen it more and more and behold, the more frequently the patient was bled, the more leeches and cupping glasses sucked out the vital fluid (for the innocent irreplaceable blood was according to him responsible for almost all ailments). In the same proportion the patient lost strength to feel pain or to express his aggravated condition by violent complaint and gestures. The patient appears more quiet in proportion as he grows weaker, the bystanders rejoice in his apparent improvement, ready to return to the same measures on the renewal of his sufferings – be they spasms, suffocation, fears or pain, for they had so beautifully quieted him before and gave promise of *further ease. In disease of long duration and when the patient retained some strength, he was deprived of food, put on a "hunger diet," in order to depress life so much more successfully and inhibit the restless states. The debilitated patient feels unable to protest against further similar measures of blood-letting leeches, vesication, warm baths and so forth to refuse their employment. That death must follow such frequently repeated reduction and exhaustion of the vital energy is not noticed by the patient, already robbed of all consciousness, and the relatives, blinded by the improvements even of the last sufferings of the patient by means of blood letting and warm baths, cannot understand and are surprised when the patient quietly slips away.*

"But God knows the patient on his bed of sickness was not treated with violence, for the prick of a small lancet is not really painful and the gum Arabic solution (Eau de Gourme, almost the only medicine that Brousseau used) was mild in taste and without apparent action – the bite of the leeches insignificant and the blood letting by the physician done quietly while the luke warm baths could only soothe, hence the disease from the very start must have been fatal, so that the patient, notwithstanding all efforts of the physician, had to leave the earth." In this way the relatives, and especially the heirs of the dear departed, consoled themselves.

The physicians in Europe and elsewhere accepted this convenient treatment of all disease according to a single rule, since it saved them from all further thinking (the most laborious of all work under the sun). They only had to take care "to assuage the pangs of conscience and console themselves that they were not the originators of this system and this method of treatment, that all the other thousands of Brousseauists did the same and that possibly everything would cease with death anyway as was taught by their master." In this way many thousand physicians were miserably misled to shed (with cold heart) the warm blood of their patients that were capable of cure and thereby rob millions of men gradually of their life, according to Brousseau's method, more than fell on Napoleon's battlefields. Was it perhaps necessary by the disposition of God for that system of Brousseau which destroyed medically the life of curable patients to precede homoeopathy in order to open the eyes of the world to the only true science and art of medicine, homoeopathy, in which curable patients find health and new life when this most difficult of all arts is practised by an indefatigable discriminating physician in a pure and conscientious manner?

[74] Only in the most urgent cases, where danger to life and imminent death allow no time for the action of a homoeopathic remedy – not hours, sometimes not even quarter-hours, and scarcely minutes – in sudden accidents occurring to previously healthy individuals – for example, in asphyxia and suspended animation from lightning, from suffocation, freezing, drowning, etc. – is it admissible and judicious, at all events as a preliminary measure to stimulate the irritability and sensibility (the physical life) with a palliative, as for instance, with gentle electrical shocks, with clysters of strong coffee, with a stimulating odor, gradual application of heat, etc. When this stimulation is effected, the play of the vital organs again goes on in its former healthy manner, for there is here no disease* to be removed, but merely an obstruction and suppression of the healthy vital force. To this category belong various antidotes to sudden poisoning: alkalies from mineral acids, hepar sulphuris for metallic poisons, coffee and camphora (and ipecacuanha) for poisoning by opium, etc.

It does not follow that a homoeopathic medicine has been ill selected for a case of disease because some of the medicinal symptoms are only antipathic to some of the less important and minor symptoms of the disease; if only the others, the stronger well-marked (characteristic), and peculiar symptoms of the disease are covered and matched by the same medicine with similarity of symptoms – that is to say, overpowered, destroyed and extinguished; the few opposite symptoms also disappear of themselves after the expiry of the term of action of the medicament, without retarding the cure in the least.

*And yet the new sect that mixes the two systems appeals (though in vain) to this observation, in order that they may have an excuse for encountering everywhere such exceptions to the general rule in diseases, and to justify their convenient employment of allopathic palliatives, and of other injurious allopathic trash besides, solely for the sake of sparing themselves the trouble of seeking for the suitable homoeopathic remedy for each case of disease – I might almost say for the sake of sparing themselves the trouble of being homoeopathic physicians, and yet wishing to appear as such. But their performances are on a par with the system they pursue; they are nothing to boast of.

[75] In the living human being no permanent neutralization of contrary or antagonistic sensations can take place, as happens with substances of opposite qualities in the chemical laboratory, where, for instance, sulphuric acid and potash unite to form a perfectly different substance, a neutral salt, which is now no longer either acid or alkali, and is not decomposed even by heat. Such amalgamations and thorough combinations to form something permanently neutral and indifferent do not, as has been said, ever take place with respect to dynamic impressions of an antagonistic nature in our sensific apparatus. Only a semblance of neutralization and mutual removal occurs in such cases at first, but the antagonistic sensations do not permanently remove one another. The tears of the mourner will be dried for but a short time by a laughable play; the jokes are, however, soon forgotten, and his tears then flow still more abundantly than before.

[76] Plain as this proposition is, it has been misunderstood, and in opposition to it some have asserted "that the palliative in its secondary action, would then be similar to the disease present, must be capable of curing just as well as a homoeopathic medicine does by its primary action." But they did not reflect that the secondary action is not a product of the medicine, but invariably of the antagonistically acting vital force of the organism; that therefore this secondary action resulting from the vital force on the employment of a palliative is a state similar to the symptoms of the disease which the palliative left uneradicated, and which the reaction of the vital force against the palliative consequently increased still more.

[77] As when in a dark dungeon, where the prisoner could with difficulty recognize objects close to him, alcohol is suddenly lighted, everything is instantly illuminated in a most consolatory manner to the unhappy wretch; but when it is extinguished, the brighter the flame was previously the blacker is the night which now envelopes him, and renders everything about him much more difficult to be seen than before.

[78] The homoeopathic physician, who does not entertain the foregone conclusion devised by the ordinary school (who have fixed upon a few names of such fevers, besides which mighty nature dare not produce any others, so as to admit of their treating these disease according to some fixed method), does not acknowledge the names goal fever, bilious fever, typhus fever, putrid fever, nervous fever or mucous fever, but treats them each according to their several peculiarities.

[79] Subsequently to the year 1801 a kind of pupura miliaris (roodvonk), which came from the West, was by physicians confounded with the scarlet fever, notwithstanding that they exhibited totally different symptoms, that the latter found its prophylatic and curative remedy in belladonna, the former in aconite, and that the former was generally merely sporadic, while the latter was invariable epidemic. Of late years it seems as if the two occasionally joined to form an eruptive fever of a peculiar kind, for which neither the one nor the other remedy, alone, will be found to be exactly homoeopathic.

[80] If the patient succumbs, the practiser of such a treatment is in the habit of pointing out to the sorrowing relatives, at the post-mortem examination, these internal organic disfigurements, which are due to his pseudo-art, but which he artfully maintains to be the original incurable disease (see my book, Die Alloopathie, ein Wort deh Warnung an Kranke jeder Art, Leipzig, bei Baumgartner [translated in Lesser Writings]). Those deceitful records, the illustrated works on pathological anatomy, exhibit the products of such lamentable bungling.

[81] The only possible case of plethora shows itself with the healthy woman, several days before her monthly period, with a feeling of a certain fullness of womb and breasts, but without inflammation.

[82] Among all imaginable methods for the relief of sickness, no greater allopathic, irrational or inappropriate one can be thought of than this Brousseauic, debilitating treatment by means of venesection and hunger diet, which for many years has spread over a large part of the earth. No intelligent man can see in it anything medical, or medically helpful, whereas real medicines, even if chosen blindly and administered to a patient, may at times prove of benefit in a given case of sickness because they may accidentally have been homoeopathic to the case. But from venesection, healthy common sense can expect nothing more than certain lessening and shortening of life. It is a sorrowful and wholly groundless fallacy that most and indeed all diseases depend on local inflammation. Even for true local inflammation, the most certain and quickest cure is found in medicines capable of taking away dynamically the arterial irritation upon which the inflammation is based and this without the least loss of fluids and strength. Local venesections, even from the affected part, only tend to increase renewed inflammation of these parts. And precisely so it is generally inappropriate, aye, murderous to take away many pounds of blood from the veins in inflammatory fevers, when a few appropriate medicines would dispel this irritated arterial state, driving the hitherto quiet blood together with the disease in a few hours without the least loss of fluids and strength. Such great loss of blood is evidently irreplaceable for the remaining continuance of life, since the organs intended by the Creator for bloodmaking have thereby become so weakened that while they may manufacture blood in the same quantity but not again of the same good quality. And how impossible is it for this imagined plethora to have been produced in such remarkable rapidity and so to drain it off by frequent venesections when yet an hour before the pulse of this heated patient (before the fever and chill stage) was so quiet. No man, no sick person has ever too much blood or too much strength. On the contrary, every sick man lacks strength, otherwise his vital energy would have prevented the development of the disease. Thus it is irrational and cruel to add to this weakened patient, a greater, indeed the most serious source of debility that can be imagined. It is a murderous malpractice irrational and cruel based on a wholly groundless and absurd theory instead of taking away his disease which is ever dynamic and only to be removed by dynamic potencies.

[83] If the patient succumbs, the practiser of such a treatment is in the habit of pointing out to the sorrowing relatives, at the post-mortem examination, these internal organic disfigurements, which are due to his pseudo-art, but which he artfully maintains to be the original incurable disease (see my book, Die Alloopathie, ein Wort deh Warnung an Kranke jeder Art, Leipzig, bei Baumgartner [translated in Lesser Writings]). Those deceitful records, the illustrated works on pathological anatomy, exhibit the products of such lamentable bungling. Deceased people from the country and those from the poor

of cities who have died without such bungling with hurtful measures are not opened up through pathological anatomy as a rule. Such corruption and deformities would not be found in their corpses. From this fact can be judged the value of the evidence drawn from these beautiful illustrations as well as of the honesty of these authors and book makers.

[84] During the flourishing years of youth and with the commencement of regular menstruation joined to a mode of life beneficial to soul, heart and body, they remain unrecognized for years. Those afflicted appeal in perfect health to their relatives and acquaintances and the disease that was received by infection or inheritance seems to have wholly disappeared. But in later years, after adverse events and conditions of life, they are sure to appear anew and develop the more rapidly and assume a more serious character in proportion as the vital principle has become disturbed by debilitating passions, worry and care, but especially when disordered by inappropriate medicinal treatment.

[85] I spent twelve years in investigating the source of this incredibly large number of chronic affections, in ascertaining and collecting certain proofs of this great truth, which had remained unknown to all former or contemporary observers, and in discovering at the same time the principal (antipsoric) remedies, which collectively are nearly a match for this thousand-headed monster of disease in all its different developments and forms. I have published my observations on this subject in the book entitled The Chronic Diseases (4 vols., Dresden, Arnold. [2nd edit., Dusseldorf, Schaub.]) before I had obtained this knowledge I could only treat the whole number of chronic diseases as isolated, individual maladies, with those medicinal substances whose pure effects had been tested on healthy persons up to that period, so that every case of chronic disease was treated by my disciples according to the group of symptoms it presented, just like an idiopathic disease, and it was often so for cured that sick mankind rejoiced at the extensive remedial treasures already amassed by the new healing art. How much greater cause is there now for rejoicing that the desired goal has been so much more nearly attained, inasmuch as the recently discovered and far more specific homoeopathic remedies for chronic affections arising from psora (properly termed antipsoric remedies) and the special instructions for their preparation and employment have been published; and from among them the true physician can now select for his curative agents those whose medicinal symptoms correspond in the most similar (homoeopathic) manner to the chronic disease he has to cure; and thus, by the employment of (antipsoric) medicines more suitable for this miasm, he is enabled to render more essential service and almost invariably to effect a perfect cure.

[86] Some of these causes that exercise a modifying influence on the transformation of psora into chronic diseases manifestly depend sometimes on the climate and the peculiar physical character of the place of abode, sometimes on the very great varieties in the physical and mental training of youth, both of which may have been neglected, delayed or carried to excess, or on their abuse in the business or conditions of life, in the matter of diet and regimen, passions, manners, habits and customs of various kinds.

[87] How many improper ambiguous names do not these works contain, under each of which are included excessively different morbid conditions, which often resemble each other in one single symptom only, as ague, jaundice, dropsy, consumption, leucorrhoea, haemorrhoids, rheumatism, apoplexy, convulsions, hysteria, hypochondriasis, melancholia, mania, quinsy, palsy, etc., which are represented as diseases of a fixed and unvarying character, and are treated, on account of their name, according to a determinate plan! How can the bestowal of such a name justify an identical medical treatment?

And if the treatment is not always to be the same, why make use of an identical name which postulates an identity of treatment? "Nihil sane in artem medicam pestiferum magis unquam irrepsit malum, quam generalia quaedam medicinam," says Huxham, a man as clear-sighted as he was estimable on account of his conscientiousness (Op. phys. med., tom. I.). And in like manner Frittze laments (Annalen, I, p.80) "that essentially different diseases are designated by the same name." Even those epidemic diseases, which undoubtedly may be propagated in every separate epidemic by a peculiar contagious principle which remains unknown to us, are designated, in the old school of medicine by particular names, just as if they were well-known fixed diseases that invariably recurred under the same form, as hospital fever, goal fever, camp fever, putrid fever, bilious fever, nervous fever, mucous fever, although each epidemic of such roving fevers exhibits itself at every occurrence as another, a new disease, such as it has never before appeared in exactly the same form, differing very much, in every instance, in its course, as well as in many of its most striking symptoms and its whole appearance. Each is so for dissimilar to all previous epidemics, whatever names they may bear, that it would be dereliction of all logical accuracy in our ideas of things were we to give to these maladies, that differ so much among themselves, one of those names we meet with in pathological writings, and treat them all medicinally in conformity with this misused name. The candid Sydenham alone perceived this, when he (Obs. med., cap. ii, De morb, epid.) insists upon the necessity of not considering any epidemic disease as having occurred before and treating it in the same way as another, since all that occur successively, be they ever so numerous, differ from one another: "Nihil quicquam (opinor,) animum universae qua patet medicinae pomoeria perlustrantem, tanta admiratione percellet, quam discolor illa et sui plane dissimilis morborum Epidemicorum facies; non tam qua varias ejusdem anni tempestates, quam qua discrepantes divewrsorum ab invicem annorum constitutiones referunt, ab iisque dependent. Quae tam aperta praedictorum morborum diversitas tum propriis ac sibi peculiaribus symptomatis, tum etiam medendi ratione, quam hi ab illis disparem prorsus sibi vendicant, satis illucescit. Ex quibus constat morbus hosce, ut ut externa quadantenus specie, er symptomatis aliquot utrisque pariter super venientibus, convenire paulo incautioribus videantur, re tamen ipsa (si bene adverteris animum), alienae admondum esse indolis, et distare ut aera lupinis."

    From all this it is clear that these useless and misused names of diseases ought to have no influence on the practice of the true physician, who knows that he has to judge of and to cure diseases, not according to the similarity of the name of a single one of their symptoms, but according to the totality of the signs of the individual state of each particular patient, whose affection it is his duty carefully to investigate, but never to give a hypothetical guess at it.

    If, however, it is deemed necessary sometimes to make use of names of diseases, in order, when talking about a patient to ordinary persons, to render ourselves intelligible in few words, we ought only to employ them as collective names, and tell them, eg., the patient has a kind of St. Vitus's dance, a kind of dropsy, a kind of typhus, a kind of ague; but (in order to do away once and for all with the mistaken notions these names give rise to) we should never say he has the St. Vitus's dance, the typhus, the dropsy, the ague, as there are certainly no disease of these and similar names of fixed unvarying character.

[88] Hence the following directions for investigating the symptoms are only partially applicable for acute diseases.

[89] Every interruption breaks the train of thought of the narrators, and all they would have said at first does not again occur to them in precisely the same manner after that.
[90] For instance the physician should not ask, Was not this or that circumstance present? He should never be guilty of making such suggestions, which tend to seduce the patient into giving a false answer and a false account of his symptoms.
[91] For example what was the character of his stools? How does he pass his water? How is it with his day and night sleep? What is the state of his disposition, his humor, his memory? How about the thirst? What sort of taste has he in his mouth? What kinds of food and drink are most relished? What are most repugnant to him? Has each its full natural taste, or some other unusual taste? How does he feel after eating or drinking? Has he anything to tell about the head, the limbs or the abdomen?
[92] For example, how often are his bowels moved? What is the exact character of the stools? Did the whitish evacuation consist of mucus or faeces? Had he or had he not pains during the evacuation? What was their exact character, and where were they seated? What did the patient vomit? Is the bad taste in the mouth putrid, or bitter, or sour, or what? before or after eating, or during the repast? At what period of the day was it worst? What is the taste of what is eructated? Does the urine only become turbid on standing, or is it turbid when first discharged? What is its color when first emitted? Of what color is the sediment? How does he behave during sleep? Does he whine, moan, talk or cry out in his sleep? Does he start during sleep? Does he snore during inspiration, or during expiration? Does he lie only on his back, or on which side? Does he cover himself well up, or can he not bear the clothes on him? Does he easily awake, or does he sleep too soundly? How often does this or that symptom occur? What is the cause that produces it each time it occurs? does it come on whilst sitting, lying, standing, or when in motion? only when fasting, or in the morning, or only in the evening, or only after a meal, or when does it usually appear? When did the rigor come on? was it merely a chilly sensation, or was he actually cold at the same time? if so, in what parts? or while feeling chilly, was he actually warm to the touch? was it merely a sensation of cold, without shivering? was he hot without redness of the face? what parts of him were hot to the touch? or did he complain of heat without being hot to the touch? How long did the chilliness last? how long the hot stage? When did the thirst come on – during the cold stage? during the heat? or previous to it? or subsequent to it? How great was the thirst, and what was the beverage desired? When did the sweat come on – at the beginning or the end of the heat? or how many hours after the heat? when asleep or when awake? How great was the sweat? was it warm or cold? on what parts? how did it smell? What does he complain of before or during the cold stage? what during the hot stage? what after it? what during or after the sweating stage?
[93] For example, how the patient behaved during the visit – whether he was morose, quarrelsome, hasty, lachrymose, anxious, despairing or sad, or hopeful, calm etc. Whether he was in a drowsy state or in any way dull of comprehension; whether he spoke hoarsely, or in a low tone, or incoherently, or how other wise did he talk? what was the color of his face and eyes, and of his skin generally? what degree of liveliness and power was there in his expression and eyes? what was the state of his tongue, his breathing, the smell from his mouth, and his hearing? were his pupils dilated or contracted? how rapidly and to what extent did they alter in the dark and in the light? what was the character of the pulse? what was the condition of the abdomen? how moist or hot, how cold or dry to the touch, was the skin of this or that part or generally? whether he lay with head thrown back, with mouth half or wholly open, with the arms placed above the head, on his back, or in what other position? what effort did he make

to raise himself? and anything else in him that may strike the physician as being remarkable.

(Added to the Sixth Edition)
In women, note the character of menstruation and other discharges, etc.

[94] Any causes of a disgraceful character, which the patient or his friends do not like to confess, at least not voluntarily, the physician must endeavor to elicit by skilfully framing his questions, or by private information. To these belong poisoning or attempted suicide, onanism, indulgence in ordinary or unnatural debauchery, excess in wine, cordials, punch and other ardent beverages, or coffee, – over-indulgence in eating generally, or in some particular food of a hurtful character, – infection with venereal disease or itch, unfortunate love, jealousy, domestic infelicity, worry, grief on account of some family misfortune, ill-usage, balked revenge, injured pride, embarrassment of a pecuniary nature, superstitious fear, – hunger, – or an imperfection in the private parts, a rupture, a prolapse, and so forth.

[95] In chronic diseases of females it is specially necessary to pay attention to pregnancy, sterility, sexual desire, accouchements, miscarriages, suckling, and the state of the menstrual discharge. With respect to the last-named more particularly, we should not neglect to ascertain if it recurs at too short intervals, or is delayed beyond the proper time, how many days it lasts, whether its flow is continuous or interrupted, what is its general quality, how dark is its color, whether there is leucorrhoea before its appearance or after its termination, but especially by what bodily or mental ailments, what sensations and pains, it is preceded, accompanied or followed; if there is leucorrhoea, what is its nature, what sensations attend its flow, in what quantity it is, and what are the conditions and occasions under which it occurs?

[96] A pure fabrication of symptoms and sufferings will never be met with in hypochondriacs, even in the most impatient of them – a comparison of the sufferings they complain of at various times when the physician gives them nothing at all, or something quite unmedical, proves this plainly; – but we must deduct something from their exaggeration, at all events ascribe the strong character of their expressions to their expressions when talking of their ailments becomes of itself an important symptom in the list of features of which the portrait of the disease is composed. The case is different with insane persons and rascally feigners of disease.

[97] The physician who has already, in the first cases, been able to choose a remedy approximating to the homoeopathic specific, will, from the subsequence cases, be enabled either to verify the suitableness of the medicine chosen, or to discover a more appropriate, the most appropriate homoeopathic remedy.

[98] The old school physician gave himself very little trouble in this matter in his mode of treatment. He would not listen to any minute detail of all the circumstances of his case by the patient; indeed, he frequently cut him short in his relation of his sufferings, in order that he might not be delayed in the rapid writing of his prescription, composed of a variety of ingredients unknown to him in their true effects. No allopathic physician, as has been said, sought to learn all the circumstances of the patient's case, and still less did he make a note in writing of them. On seeing the patient again several days afterwards he recollected nothing concerning the few details he had heard at the first visit (having in the meantime seen so many other patients laboring under different affections); he had allowed everything to go in at one ear and out at the other. At subsequent visits he only asked a few general questions, went through the ceremony of feeling the pulse at the wrist, looked at the tongue, and at the same moment wrote another prescription, on equally irrational principles, or ordered the first one to be continued (in considerable quantities several times a day), and, with a graceful bow, he hurried off to the fiftieth or sixtieth patient he had to visit, in this thoughtless way, in the course of that forenoon. The profession which of all others requires actually the most reflection, a conscientious, careful examination of the state of each individual patient and a special treatment founded thereon, was conducted in this manner by persons who called themselves physicians, rational practitioners. The result, as might naturally be expected, was almost invariably bad; and yet patients had to go to them for advise, partly because there were none better to be had, partly for fashion's sake.

[99] Not one single physician, as far as I know, during the previous two thousand five hundred years, thought of this so natural, so absolutely necessary and only genuine mode of testing medicines for their pure and peculiar effects in deranging the health of man, in order to learn what morbid state each medicine is capable of curing, except the great and immoral Albrecht von Haller. He alone, besides myself, saw the necessity of this (vide the Preface to the Pharmacopoeia Helvet, Basil, 1771, fol., p.12); Nempe primum in corpore sano medela tentanda est, sine peregrina ulla miscela; odoreque et sapore ejus exploratis, exigua illiu dosis ingerenda et ad ommes, quae inde contingunt, affectiones, quis pulsus, qui calor, quae respiratia, quaenam excretiones, attendum. Inde ad ductum phaenomenorum, in sano obviorum, transeas ad experimenta in corpore aegroro," etc. But no one, not a single physician, attended to or followed up this invaluable hint.

[100] It is impossible that there can be another true, best method of curing dynamic diseases (i.e., all diseases not strictly surgical) besides homoeopathy, just as it is impossible to draw more than one straight line betwixt two given points. He who imagines that there are other modes of curing diseases besides it could not have appreciated homoeopathy fundamentally nor practised it with sufficient care, nor could he ever have seen or read cases of properly performed homoeopathic cures; nor, on the other hand, could he have discerned the baselessness of all allopathic modes of treating diseases and their bad or even dreadful effects, if, with such lax indifference, he places the only true healing art on an equality with those hurtful methods of treatment, or alleges the latter to be auxiliaries to homoeopathy which it could not do without! My true, conscientious followers, the pure homoeopathists, with their successful, almost never-failing treatment, might teach these persons better.

[101] The first fruits of these labors, as perfect as they could be at that time, I recorded in the Fragmenta de viribus medicamentorum positivis, sive in sano corpore humano observatis, pts. I, ii, Lipsiae, 8, 1805, ap. J. A. Barth; the more mature fruits in the Reine Arzneimittellebre, I Th., dritte Ausg.; II Th., dritte Ausg., 1833; III Th., zweite Ausg., 1825; IV Th., zw. Ausg., 1827 (English translation, Materia Medica Pura, vols I and ii); and in the second, third, and fourth parts of Die chronischen Krankheiten, 1828, 1830, Dresden bei Arnold (2nd edit., with a fifth part, Dusseldorf bei Schaub, 1835, 1839).

[102] See what I have said on this subject in the "Examination of the Sources of the Ordinary Materia Medica," prefixed to the third part of my Reine Arzneimittellebre (translated in the Materia Medica Pura, vol. ii).

[103] Some few persons are apt to faint from the smell of roses and to fall into many other morbid, and sometimes dangerous states from partaking of mussels, crabs or the roe of the barbel, from touching the leaves of some kinds of sumach, etc.

[104] Thus the Princess Maria Porphyroghnita restored her brother, the Emperor Alexius, who suffered from faintings, by sprinkling him with rose water in the presence of his aunt Eudoxia (Hist. byz. Alexias, lib. xv, p. 503, ed. Posser); and Horstius (Oper., iii, p.59) saw great benefit from rose vinegar in cases of syncope.

[105] This fact was also perceived by the estimable A. v. Haller, who says (Preface to his Hist. stirp. helv.): "Latet immensa virium diversitas in iis ipsis plantis, quarum facies externas dudum novimus, animas quasi et quodcunque caelestius habent, nondum perspeximus."

[106] Anyone who has a thorough knowledge of, and can appreciate the remarkable difference of, effects on the health of man of every single substance from those of every other, will readily perceive that among them there can be, in a medical point of view, no equivalent remedies whatever, no surrogates. Only those who do not know the pure, positive effects of the different medicines can be so foolish as to try to persuade us that one can serve in the stead of the other, and can in the same disease prove just as serviceable as the other. Thus do ignorant children confound the most essential different things, because they scarcely know their external appearances, far less their real value, their true importance and their very dissimilar inherent properties.

[107] If this be pure truth, as it undoubtedly is, then no physician who would not be regarded as devoid of reason, and who would not act contrary to the dictates of his conscience, the sole arbiter of real worth, can employ in the treatment of diseases any medicinal substance but one with whose real significance he is thoroughly and perfectly conversant, i.e., whose positive action on the health of healthy individuals he has so accurately tested that he knows for certain that it is capable of producing a very similar morbid state, more similar than any other medicine with which he is perfectly acquainted, to that presented by the case of disease he intends to cure by means of it; for, as has been shown above, neither man, nor mighty Nature herself, can effect a perfect, rapid and permanent cure otherwise than with a homoeopathic remedy. Henceforth no true physician can abstain from making such experiment, in order to obtain this most necessary and only knowledge of the medicines that are essential to cure, this knowledge which has hitherto been neglected by the physicians in all ages. In all former ages – posterity will scarcely believe it – physicians have hitherto contented themselves with blindly prescribing for diseases medicines whose value was unknown, and which had never been tested relative to their highly important, very various, pure dynamic action on the health of man; and, moreover, they mingled several of these unknown medicines that differed so vastly among each other in one formula, and left it to chance to determine what effects should thereby be produced on the patient. This is just as if a madman should force his way into the workshop of an artisan, seize upon handfuls of very different tools, with the uses of all of which he is quite unacquainted, in order, as he imagines, to work at the objects of art he sees around him. I need hardly remark that these would be destroyed, I may say utterly ruined, by his senseless operations.

[108] Young green peas, green French beans ('boiled potatoes' in the Sixth Edition) and in all cases carrots are allowable, as the least medicinal vegetables.

[109] The subject of experiment must either be not in the habit of taking pure wine, brandy, coffee or tea, or he must have totally abstained for a considerable time previously from the use of these injurious beverages, some of which are stimulating, others medicinal.

[110] He who makes known to the medical world the results of such experiments becomes thereby responsible for the trustworthiness of the person experimented on and his statements, and justly so, as the weal of suffering humanity is here at stake.

[111] Those trials made by the physician on himself have for him other and inestimable advantages. In the first place, the great truth that the medicinal virtue of all drugs, whereon depends their curative power, lies in the changes of health he has himself undergone from the medicines he has proved, and the morbid states he has himself experi-

enced from them, becomes for him an incontrovertible fact. Again by such noteworthy observations on himself he will be brought to understand his own sensations, his mode of thinking and his disposition (the foundation of all true wisdom), and he will be also trained to be, what every physician ought to be, a good observer. All our observations on others are not nearly so interesting as those made on ourselves. The observer of others must always dread lest the experimenter did not feel exactly what he said, or lest he did not describe his sensations with the most appropriate expressions. He must always remain in doubt whether he has not been deceived, at least to some extent. These obstacles to the knowledge of the truth, which can never be thoroughly surmounted in our investigations of the artificial morbid symptoms that occur in others from the ingestion of medicines, cease entirely when we make the trials on ourselves. He who makes these trials on himself knows for certain what he has felt, and each trial is a new inducement for him to investigate the powers of other medicines. He thus becomes more and more practised in the art of observing, of such importance to the physician, by continuing to observe himself, the one on whom he can most rely and who will never deceive him; and this he will do all the more zealously as these experiments on himself promise to give him a reliable knowledge of the true value and significance of the instruments of cure that are still to a great degree unknown to our art. Let it not be imagined that such slight indispositions caused by taking medicines for the purpose of proving them can be in the main injurious to the health. Experience shows on the contrary, that the organism of the prover becomes, by these frequent attacks on his health, all the more expert in repelling all external influences inimical to his frame and all artificial and natural morbific noxious agents, and becomes more hardened to resist everything of an injurious character, by means of these moderate experiments on his own person with medicines. His health becomes more unalterable; he becomes more robust, as all experience shows.

[112] Symptoms which, during the whole course of the disease, might have been observed only a long time previously, or never before, consequently new ones, belonging to the medicine.

[113] Latterly it has been the habit to entrust the proving of medicines to unknown persons at a distance, who were paid for their work, and the formation so obtained was printed. But by so doing, the work which is of all others the most important, which is to form the basis of the only true healing art, and which demands the greatest moral certainty and trustworthiness seems to me, I regret to say, to become doubtful and uncertain in its results and to lose all value.

[114] At first, I was the only person who made the provings of the pure powders of medicines the most important of his occupations. Since then I have been assisted in this by some young men, who instituted experiments on themselves, and whose observations I have critically revised. Following these some genuine work of this kind was done by a few others. But what shall we not be able to effect in the way of curing in the whole extent of the infinitely large domain of disease, when numbers of accurate and trustworthy observers shall have rendered their services in enriching this, the only true materia medica, by careful experiments on themselves! The healing art will then come near the mathematical sciences in certainty.

[115] See the second note to §109.

[116] At first, about forty years ago, I was the only person who made the provings of the pure powders of medicines the most important of his occupations. Since then I have been assisted in this by some young men, who instituted experiments on themselves, and whose observations I have critically revised. Following these some genuine work of this

kind was done by a few others. But what shall we not be able to effect in the way of curing in the whole extent of the infinitely large domain of disease, when numbers of accurate and trustworthy observers shall have rendered their services in enriching this, the only true materia medica, by careful experiments on themselves! The healing art will then come near the mathematical sciences in certainty.

[117] But this laborious, sometimes very laborious, search for and selection of the homoeopathic remedy most suitable in every respect to each morbid state, is an operation which, notwithstanding all the admirable books for facilitating it, still demands the study of the original sources themselves, and at the same time a great amount of circumspection and serious deliberation, which have their best rewards in the consciousness of having faithfully discharged our duty. How could his laborious, care-demanding task, by which alone the best way of curing diseases is rendered possible, please the gentlemen of the new mongrel sect, who assume the honorable name of homoeopathists, and even seem to employ medicines in form and appearance homoeopathic, but determined upon by them anyhow (quidquid in buccam venit), and who, when the unsuitable remedy does not immediately give relief, in place of laying the blame on their unpardonable ignorance and laxity in performing the most and important and serious of all human affairs, ascribe it to homoeopathy, which they accuse of great imperfection (if the truth be told, its imperfection consists in this, that the most suitable homoeopathic remedy for each morbid condition does not spontaneously fly into their mouths like roasted pigeons, without any trouble on their own part). They know, however, from frequent practice, how to make up for the inefficiency of the scarcely half homoeopathic remedy by the employment of allopathic means, that come much more handy to them, among which one or more dozens of leeches applied to the affected part, or little harmless venesections to the extent of eight ounces, and so forth, play an important part; and should the patient, in spite of all this, recover, they extol their venesections, leeches, etc., alleging that, had it not been for these, the patient would not have been pulled through, and they give us to understand, in no doubtful language, that these operations, derived without much exercise of genius from the pernicious routine of the old school, in reality contributed the best share towards the cure. But if the patient die under the treatment, as not unfrequently happens, they seek to console the friends by saying that "they themselves were witnesses that everything conceivable had been done for the lamented deceased". Who would do this frivolous and pernicious tribe the honour to call them, after the name of the very laborious but salutary art, homoeopathic physicians? May the just recompense await them, that, when taken ill, they may be treated in the same manner!

[118] Dr. von Bonninghausen, who has already distinguished himself by his labours in connection with the new system of medicine, has lately increased our obligation to him by the publication of his important little book setting forth the characteristic symptoms, more particularly of the antipsoric medicines, entitled Uebersicht der Hauptwirkungs-Sphure der antips. Arz., Munster, bei Coppenrath, 1883, and the appendix thereto (containing the antisyphilitic and the antisycotic medicines) at the end of the second edition of his Systematisch-alphabetisches Repertorium der antipsorischen Arzneien, bei Coppenrath in Munster.

[119] Dr. von Bonninghausen, by the publication of the characteristic symptoms of homoeopathic medicines and his repertory has rendered a great service to Homoeopathy as well as Dr. J.H.G. Jahr in his handbook of principal symptoms.

[120] This exaltation of the medicinal symptoms over those disease symptoms analogous to them, which looks like an aggravation, has been observed by other physicians also, when by accident they employed a homoeopathic remedy. When a patient suffering from itch complains of an increase of the eruption after sulphur, his physician who knows not the cause of this, consoles him with the assurance that the itch must first come out properly before it can be cured; he knows not, however, that this is a sulphur eruption, that assumes the appearance of an increase of the itch.

"The facial eruption which the viola tricolor cured was aggravated by it at the commencement of its action," Leroy tells us (Heilk, fur Mutter, p.406), but he knew not that the apparent aggravation was owing to the somewhat too large dose of the remedy, which in this instance was to a certain extent homoeopathic. Lysons says (Med. Transact., vol ii, London, 1772), "The bark of the elm cures most certainly those skin diseases which it increases at the beginning of its action." Had he not given the bark in the monstrous doses usual in the allopathic system, but in the quite small doses requisite when the medicine shows similarity of symptoms, that is to say, when it is used homoeopathically, he would have effected a cure without, or almost without, seeing this apparent increase of the disease (homoeopathic aggravation).

[121] When they were not caused by an important error in regimen, a violent emotion, or a tumultuous revolution in the organism, such as the occurrence or cessation of the menses, conception, childbirth, and so forth.

[122] In cases where the patient (which, however, happens excessively seldom in chronic, but not infrequently in acute, diseases) feels very ill, although his symptoms are very indistinct, so that this state may be attributed more to the benumbed state of the nerves, which does not permit the patient's pains and sufferings to be distinctly perceived, this torpor of the internal sensibility is removed by opium, and in its secondary action the symptoms of the disease become distinctly apparent.

[123] One of the many great and pernicious blunders of the old school.

[124] Foot-note in Fifth Edition only.
   As, for instance, aconite, rhus, belladonna, mercury, etc.

[125] Recent itch eruption, chancre, condylomata.

[126] Recent itch eruption, chancre, condylomata, as I have indicated in my book of Chronic Diseases.

[127] As was the case before my time with the remedies for the condylomatous disease (and the antipsoric medicines).

[128] The issues of the old-school do something similar; as artificial ulcers on external parts, they silence some internal chronic diseases, but only for a short time, without being able to cure them; but, on the other hand, they weaken and destroy the general health much more than is done by most of the metastases effected by the instinctive vital force.

[129] The issues of the old-school do something similar; as artificial ulcers on external parts, they silence some internal chronic diseases, but only for a short time, as long as they cause a painful irritation to which the sick organism is not used, without being able to cure them; but, on the other hand, they weaken and destroy the general health much more than is done by most of the metastases effected by the instinctive vital force.

[130] For any medicines that might at the same time be given internally served but to aggravate the malady, as these remedies possessed no specific power of curing the whole disease, but assailed the organism, weakened it and inflicted on it, in addition, other chronic medicinal diseases.

[131] I cannot therefore advise, for instance, the local extirpation of the so-called cancer of the lips and face by means of the arsenical remedy of Frere Cosme, not only because it is excessively painful and often fails, but more for this reason, because, if this dynamic remedy should indeed succeed in freeing the affected part of the body from the

malignant ulcer locally, the basic malady is thereby not diminished in the slightest, the preserving vital force is therefore necessitated to transfer the field of operation of the great internal malady to some more important part (as it does in every case of metastasis), and the consequence is blindness, deafness, insanity, suffocative asthma, dropsy, apoplexy, etc. But this ambiguous local liberation of the part from the malignant ulcer by the topical arsenical remedy only succeeds, after all, in those cases where the ulcer has not yet attained any great size, and when the vital force is still very energetic; but it is just in such a state of things that the complete internal cure of the whole original disease is also still practicable.

The result is the same without previous cure of the inner miasm when cancer of the face or breast is removed by the knife alone and when encysted tumors are enucleated; something worse ensues, or at any rate death is hastened. This has been the case times without number, but the old school still goes blindly on in the same way in every new case, with the same disastrous results.

[132] Itch eruption, chancre (bubo), condylomata.

[133] I cannot therefore advise, for instance, the local extirpation of the so-called cancer of the lips and face (the product of highly developed psora, not infrequently in conjunction with syphilis) by means of the arsenical remedy of Frere Cosme, not only because it is excessively painful and often fails, but more for this reason, because, if this dynamic remedy should indeed succeed in freeing the affected part of the body from the malignant ulcer locally, the basic malady is thereby not diminished in the slightest, the preserving vital force is therefore necessitated to transfer the field of operation of the great internal malady to some more important part (as it does in every case of metastasis), and the consequence is blindness, deafness, insanity, suffocative asthma, dropsy, apoplexy, etc. But this ambiguous local liberation of the part from the malignant ulcer by the topical arsenical remedy only succeeds, after all, in those cases where the ulcer has not yet attained any great size, and when the vital force is still very energetic; but it is just in such a state of things that the complete internal cure of the whole original disease is also still practicable.

The result is the same without previous cure of the inner miasm when cancer of the face or breast is removed by the knife alone and when encysted tumors are enucleated; something worse ensues, or at any rate death is hastened. This has been the case times without number, but the old school still goes blindly on in the same way in every new case, with the same disastrous results.

[134] In investigations of this nature we must not allow ourselves to be deceived by the assertions of the patients of their friends, who frequently assign as the cause of chronic, even of the severest and most inveterate diseases, either a cold caught (a thorough wetting, drinking cold water after being heated) many years ago, or a former fright, a sprain, a vexation (sometimes even a bewitchment), etc. These causes are much too insignificant to develop a chronic disease in a healthy body, to keep it up for years, and to aggravate it year by year, as is the case with all chronic diseases from developed psora. Causes of a much more important character than those remembered noxious influences must lie at the root of the initiation and progress of a serious, obstinate disease of long standing; the assigned causes could only rouse into activity the latent chronic miasm.

[135] In investigations of this nature we must not allow ourselves to be deceived by the assertions of the patients of their friends, who frequently assign as the cause of chronic, even of the severest and most inveterate diseases, either a cold caught (a thorough wetting, drinking cold water after being heated) many years ago, or a former fright, a

sprain, a vexation (sometimes even a bewitchment), etc. These causes are much too insignificant to develop a chronic disease in a healthy body, to keep it up for years, and to aggravate it year by year, as is the case with all chronic diseases from developed psora. Causes of a much more important character than those remembered noxious influences must lie at the root of the initiation and progress of a serious, obstinate disease of long standing; the assigned causes could only rouse into activity the latent chronic miasm.

[136] *How often, for instance, do we not meet with a mild, soft disposition in patients who have for years been afflicted with the most painful diseases, so that the physician feels constrained to esteem and compassionate the sufferer! But if he subdue the disease and restore the patient to health – as is frequently done in homoeopathic practice – he is often astonished and horrified at the frightful alteration in his disposition. He often witnesses the occurrence of ingratitude, cruelty, refined malice and propensities most disgraceful and degrading to humanity, which were precisely the qualities possessed by the patient before he grew ill.*

Those who were patient when well often become obstinate, violent, hasty, or even intolerant and capricious, or impatient or disponding when ill; those formerly chaste and modest often frequently become lascivious and shameless. A clear-headed person not infrequently becomes obtuse of intellect, while one ordinarily weak-minded becomes more prudent and thoughtful; and a man slow to make up his mind sometimes acquires great presence of mind and quickness of resolve, etc.

[137] *Thus aconite will seldom or never effect a rapid or permanent cure in a patient of a quiet, calm, equable disposition; and just as little will nux vomica be serviceable where the disposition is mild and phlegmatic, pulsatilla where it is happy, gay and obstinate, or ignatia where it is imperturbable and disposed neither to be frightened nor vexed.*

[138] *It very rarely happens that a mental or emotional disease of long standing ceases spontaneously (for the internal dyscrasia transfers itself again to the grosser corporeal organs); such are the few cases met with now and then, where a former inmate of a madhouse has been dismissed apparently recovered. Hitherto, moreover, all madhouses have continued to be chokefull, so that the multitude of other insane persons who seek for admission into such institutions could scarcely find room in them unless some of the insane in the house died. Not one is ever really and permanently cured in them! A convincing proof, among many others, of the complete nullity of the non-healing art hitherto practised, which has been ridiculously honored by allopathic ostentation with the title of rational medicine. How often, on the other hand, has not the true healing art, genuine pure homoeopathy, been able to restore such unfortunate beings to the possession of their mental and corporeal health, and so give them back again to their delighted friends and to the world!*

[139] *It would seem as though the mind, in these cases, felt with uneasiness and grief the truth of these rational representations and acted upon the body as it wished to restore the lost harmony, but that the body, by means of its disease, reacted upon the organs of the mind and disposition and put them in still greater disorder by a fresh transference of its sufferings on to them.*

[140] *It is impossible to marvel at the hard-heartedness and indiscretion of the medical men in many establishments for patients of this kind, who, without attempting to discover the true and only efficacious mode of curing such disease, which is by homoeopathic medicinal (antipsoric) means, content themselves with torturing these most pitiable of all human beings with the most violent blows and other painful torments. By this*

unconscientious and revolting procedure they debase themselves beneath the level of the turnkeys in a house of correction, for the latter inflict such chastisement as the duty devolving on their office, and on criminals only, whilst the former appear, from a humiliating consciousness of their uselessness as physicians, only to vent their spite at the supposed incurability of mental diseases in harshness towards the pitiable, innocent sufferers, for they are too ignorant to be of any use and too indolent to adopt a judicious mode of treatment.

[141] Foot-note in Sixth Edition only.

The treatment of the violent insane manic and melancholic can take place only in an institution specially arranged for their treatment but not within the family circle of the patient.

[142] Two or three states may alternate with one another. Thus, for instance, in the case of double alternating diseases, certain pains may occur persistently in the legs, etc., immediately on the disappearance of a kind of ophthalmia, which latter again appears as soon as the pain in the limbs has gone off for the time – convulsions and spasms may alternate immediately with any other affection of the body or some part of it – in a case of threefold alternating states in a common indisposition, periods of apparent increase of health and unusual exaltation of the corporeal and mental powers (extravagant gaiety, extraordinary activity of the body, excess of comfortable feeling, inordinate appetite, etc.) may occur, after which, and quite unexpectedly, gloomy, melancholy humor, intolerable hypochondriacal derangement of the disposition, with disorder of several of the vital operations, the digestion, sleep, etc., appear, which again, and just as suddenly, give place to the habitual moderate ill-health; and so also several and very various alternating states. When the new state makes its appearance, there is often no perceptible trace of the former one. In other cases only slight traces of the former alternating state remain when the new one occurs; few of the symptoms of the first state remain on the appearance and during the continuance of the second. Sometimes the morbid alternating states are quite of opposite natures, as for instance, melancholy periodically alternating with gay insanity or frenzy.

[143] The pathology hitherto in vogue, which is still in the stage of irrational infancy, recognizes but one single intermittent fever, which it likewise termed ague, and admits of no varieties but such as are constituted by the different intervals at which the paroxysms recur, quotidian, tertian, quartan etc. But there are much more important differences among them than what are marked by the periods of their recurrence; there are innumerable varieties of these fevers, some of which cannot even be denominated ague, as their fits consist solely of heat; others, again, are characterised by cold alone, with or without subsequent perspiration; yet others which exhibit general coldness of the surface, with a sensation on the patient's part, or whilst the body feels externally hot, the patient feels cold; others, again, in which one paroxysm consists entirely of a rigor or simple chilliness followed by an interval of health, while the next consists of heat alone, followed or not by perspiration; others, again, in which the heat comes first and the cold stage not till that is gone; others, again, wherein after a cold or hot stage apyrexia ensues, and then perspiration comes on like a second fit, often many hours subsequently; others, again, in which no perspiration at all comes on, and yet others in which the whole attack consists of perspiration alone, without any cold or hot stage, or in which the perspiration is only present during the heat; and there are innumerable other differences, especially in regard to the accessory symptoms, such as headache of a peculiar kind, bad taste of the mouth, nausea, vomiting, diarrhoea, want of or excessive thirst, peculiar pains in the body or limbs, disturbed sleep, deliria, alterations of temper,

spasms, etc., before, during or after the sweating stage, and countless other varieties. All these are manifestly intermittent fevers of very different kinds, each of which, as might naturally be supposed, requires a special (homoeopathic) treatment. It must be confessed that they can almost all be suppressed (as is often done) by enormous doses of bark and of its pharmaceutical preparation, the sulphate of quinine; that is to say, their periodical recurrence (their typus) may be extinguished by it, but the patients who suffered from intermittent fevers for which cinchona bark is not suitable, as is the case with all those epidemic intermittent fevers that traverse whole countries and even mountainous districts, are not restored to health by the extinction of the typus; on the contrary, they now remain ill in another manner, and worse, often much worse, than before; they are affected by peculiar, chronic bark dyscrasias, and can scarcely be restored to health even by a prolonged treatment by the true system of medicine – and yet that is what is called curing, forsooth!

[144] Dr. von Bonninghausen, who has rendered more services to our beneficent system of medicine than any other of my disciples, has best elucidated this subject, which demands so much care, and has facilitated the choice of the efficient remedy for the various epidemics of fever, in his work entitled Versuch einer homoopathischen Therapie der Wechselfieber, 1833, Muster bi Regensberg.

[145] This is observed in the fatal cases, by no means rare, in which a moderate dose of opium given during the cold stage quickly deprived the patients of life.

[146] Large, oft-repeated doses of cinchona bark, as also concentrated cinchona remedies, such as the sulphate of quinine, have certainly the power of freeing such patients from the periodical fits of the marsh ague; but those thus deceived into the belief that they are cured remain diseased in another way.

[147] Large, oft-repeated doses of cinchona bark, as also concentrated cinchona remedies, such as the sulphate of quinine, have certainly the power of freeing such patients from the periodical fits of the marsh ague; but those thus deceived into the belief that they are cured remain diseased in another way, frequently with an incurable Quinin intoxication (see §276 note.)

[148] In the former editions of the Organon I have advised that a single dose of a well-selected homoeopathic medicine should always be allowed first fully to expend its action before a new medicine is given or the same one repeated – a doctrine which was the result of the positive experience that neither by a larger dose of the remedy, which may have been well chosen (as has been again recently proposed, but which would be very like a retrograde movement), nor, what amounts to the same thing, by several doses of it given in quick succession, can the greatest possible good be effected in the treatment of diseases, more especially of chronic ones; and the reason of this is, that by such a procedure the vital force dose not quietly adapt itself to the transition from the natural disease to the similar medicinal disease, but is usually so violently excited and disturbed by a larger dose, or by smaller doses of even a homoeopathically chosen remedy given rapidly one after the other, that in most cases its reaction will be anything but salutary and will do more harm than good. As long as no more efficacious mode of proceeding than that then taught by me was discovered, the safe philanthropic maxim of sin non juvat, modo ne noceat, rendered it imperative for the homoeopathic practitioner, for whom the weal of his fellow-creatures was the highest object, to allow, as a general rule in diseases, but a single dose at a time, and that the very smallest, of the carefully selected remedy to act upon the patient and, moreover, to exhaust its action. The very smallest, I repeat, for it holds good and will continue to hold good as a homoeopathic therapeutic maxim not to be refuted by any experience in the world, that the best

doses of the properly selected remedy is always the very smallest on in one of the high potencies (X), as well for chronic as for acute as for acute diseases – a truth that is the inestimable property of pure homoeopathy and which as long as allopathy and the new mongrel sect, whose treatment is a mixture of allopathic and homoeopathic processes is not much better continues to gnaw like a cancer at the life of sick human beings, and to ruin them by large and ever larger doses of drugs, will keep pure homoeopathy separated from these spurious arts as by an impassable gulf.

On the other hand, however, practice shows us that though a single one of these small doses may suffice to accomplish almost all that it was possible for this medicine to do under the circumstances, in some, and especially in slight cases of disease, particularly in those of young children and very delicate and excitable adults, yet that in many, indeed in most cases, not only of very chronic diseases that have already made great progress and have frequently been aggravated by a previous employment of inappropriate medicines, but also of serious acute diseases, one such smallest dose of medicine in our highly potentized dynamization is evidently insufficient to effect all the curative action that might be expected from that medicine, for it may unquestionably be requisite to administer several of them, in order that the vital force may be pathogenetically altered by them to such a degree and its salutary reaction stimulated to such a height, as to enable it to completely extinguish, by its reaction, the whole of that portion of the original disease that it lay in the power of the well-selected homoeopathic remedy to eradicate; the best chosen medicine in such a small dose, given but once, might certainly be of some service, but would not be nearly sufficient.

But the careful homoeopathic physician would not venture soon to repeat the same dose of the same remedy again, as from such a practice he has frequently experienced no advantage, but most frequently, on close observation, decided disadvantage. He generally witnessed aggravation, from even the smallest dose of the most suitable remedy, which he has given one day, when he repeated the next day and the next.

Now, in cases where he was convinced of the correctness of his choice of the homoeopathic medicine, in order to obtain more benefit for the patient than he was able to get hitherto from prescribing a single small dose, the idea often naturally struck him to increase the dose, since, for the reason given above, one single dose only should be given; an, for instance, in place of giving a single very minute globule moistened with the medicine in the highest dynamization, to administer six, seven or eight of them at once, and even a half or a whole drop. But the result was almost always less favourable than it should have been; it was often actually unfavourable, often even very bad – an injury that, in a patient so treated, is difficult to repair.

The difficulty in this case is not solved by giving, instead, lower dynamizations of the remedy in a large dose.

Thus, increasing the strength of the single doses of the homoeopathic medicine with the view of effecting the degree of pathogenic excitation of the vital force necessary to produce satisfactory salutary reaction, fails altogether, as experience teaches, to accomplish the desired object. This vital force is thereby too violent and too suddenly assailed and excited to allow it time to exercise a gradual equable, salutary reaction, to adapt itself to the modification effected in it; hence it strives to repel, as if it were an enemy, the medicine attacking it in excessive force, by means of vomiting, diarrhoea, fever, perspiration, and so forth, and thus in a great measure it diverts and renders nugatory the aim of the incautious physician – little or no good towards curing the disease will be thereby accomplished; on the contrary, the patient will be thereby perceptibly weakened and, for a long time, the administration of even the smallest dose of the same remedy must not be thought of if we would not wish it to injure the patient.

But it happens, moreover, that a number of the smallest doses given for the same object in quick succession accumulate in the organism into a kind of excessively large dose, with (a few cases excepted) similar bad results; in this case the vital force, not being able to recover itself betwixt every dose, though it be but small, becomes oppressed and overwhelmed, and thus being incapable of reacting in a salutary manner, it is necessitated passively to allow involuntary the continuance of the over-strong medicinal disease that has thus been forced upon it, just in the same manner as we may every day observe from the allopathic abuse of large cumulative doses of one and the same medicine, to the lasting injury of the patient.

Now, therefore, in order, whilst avoiding the erroneous method I have here pointed out, to attain the desired object more certainly than hitherto, and to administer the medicine selected in such a manner that it must exercise all its efficacy without injury to the patient, that it may effect all the good it is capable of performing in a given case of disease, I have lately adopted a particular method.

I perceived that, in order to discover this true middle path, we must be guided as well by the nature of the different medicinal substances, as also by the corporeal constitution of the patient and the magnitude of the disease, so that – to give an example from the use of sulphur in chronic (psoric) diseases – the smallest dose of it (tinct, sulph. X?) can seldom be repeated with advantage, seen in the most robust patients and in fully developed psora, oftener than every seven days, a period of time which must be proportionally lengthened when we have to treat weaker and more excitable patients of this kind; in such cases we would do well to give such a dose only every nine, twelve, or fourteen days, and continue to repeat the medicine until it ceases to be of service. We thus find (to abide by the instance of sulphur) that in sporic diseases seldom fewer than four, often however, six, eight and even ten doses (tinct. sulph. X?) are required to be successively administered at these intervals for the complete annihilation of the whole portion of the chronic disease that is eradicated by sulphur – provided always there had been no previous allopathic abuse of sulphur in the case. Thus even a (primary) scabious eruption of recent origin, though it may have spread all over the body, may be perfectly cured, in persons who are not too weakly, by a dose of tinct sulph. X? given every seven days, in the course of from ten to twelve weeks (accordingly with ten or twelve such globules), so that it will seldom be necessary to aid the cure with a few doses of carb. veg. X? (also given at the rate of one dose per week) without the slightest external treatment besides frequent changes of linen and good regimen.

When for other serious chronic diseases also we may consider it requisite, as far as we can calculate, to give eight, nine or ten doses of tinct. sulph. (at X?) it is yet more expedient in such cases, instead of giving them in uninterrupted succession, to interpose after every, or every second or third dose, a dose of another medicine, which in this case is next in point of homoeopathic suitableness to sulphur (usually hep. sulph.) and to allow this likewise to act for eight, nine, twelve or fourteen days before again commencing a course of three doses of sulphur.

But it not infrequently happens that the vital force refuses to permit several doses of sulphur, even though they may be essential for the cure of the chronic malady and are given at the intervals mentioned above, to act quietly on itself; this refusal it reveals by some, though moderate, sulphur symptoms, which it allows to appear in the patient during the treatment. In such cases it is sometimes advisable to administer a small dose of nux vom. X?, allowing it to act for eight or ten days, in order to dispose the system again to allow succeeding doses of the sulphur to act quietly and effectually upon it. In those cases for which it is adapted, puls. X? is preferable.

But the vital force shows the greatest resistance to the salutary action upon itself of the strongly indicated sulphur, and even exhibits manifest aggravation of the chronic disease, though the sulphur be given in the very smallest dose, though only a globule of the size of a mustard seed moistened with tinct. sulph X? be smelt, if the sulphur have formerly (it may be years since) been improperly given allopathically in large doses. This is one lamentable circumstance that renders the best medical treatment of chronic disease almost impossible among the many that the ordinary bungling treatment of chronic diseases by the old school would leave us nothing to do but to deplore, were there not some mode of getting over the difficulty.

In such cases we have only to let the patient smell a single time strongly at a globule the size of a mustard seed moistened with mercur metall. X, and allow this olfaction to act for about nine days, in order to make the vital force again disposed to permit the sulphur (at least the olfaction of tinct. sulph. X?) to exercise a beneficial influence on itself – a discovery for which we are indepted to Dr. Griesselich, of Carlsruhe.

[148b] What I said in the fifth edition of the organon, in a long note to this paragraph in order to prevent these undesirable reactions of the vital energy, was all the experience I then had justified. But during the last four or five years, however, all these difficulties are wholly solved by my new altered but perfected method. The same carefully selected medicine may now be given daily and for months, if necessary in this way, namely, after the lower degree of potency has been used for one or two weeks in the treatment of chronic disease, advance is made in the same way to higher degrees, (beginning according to the new dynamization method, taught herewith with the use of the lowest degrees).

[149] We ought not even with the best chosen homoeopathic medicine, for instance one pellet of the same potency that was beneficial at first, to let the patient have a second or third dose, taken dry. In the same way, if the medicine was dissolved in water and the first dose proved beneficial, a second or third and even smaller dose from the bottle standing undisturbed, even in intervals of a few days, would prove no longer beneficial, even though the original preparation had been potentized with ten succussions or as I suggested later with but two succussions in order to obviate this disadvantage and this according to above reasons. But through modification of every dose in its dynamiztion degree, as I herewith teach, there exists no offence, even if the doses be repeated more frequently, even if the medicine be ever so highly potentized with ever so many succussions. It almost seems as if the best selected homoeopathic remedy could best extract the morbid disorder from the vital force and in chronic disease to extinguish the same only if applied in several different forms.

[150] Made in 40, 30, 20, 15 or 8 tablespoons of water with the addition of some alcohol or a piece of charcoal in order to preserve it. If charcoal is used, it is suspended by means of a thread in the vial and is taken out when the vial is succussed. The solution of the medicinal globule (and it is rarely necessary to use more than one globule) of a thoroughly potentized medicine in a large quantity of water can be obviated by making a solution in only 7-8 tablespoons of water and after thorough succussion of the vial take from it one tablespoon and put it in a glass of water (containing about 7 to 8 spoonfuls), this stirred thoroughly and then given a dose to the patient. If he is unusually excited and sensitive, a teaspoon of this solution may be put in a second glass of water, thoroughly stirred and teaspoonful doses or more be given. There are patients of so great sensitiveness that a third or fourth glass, similarly prepared, may be necessary.

Each such prepared glass must be made fresh daily. the globule of the high potency is best crushed in a few grains of sugar of milk which the patient can put in the vial and be dissolved in the requisite quantity of water.

[151] As all experience shows that the dose of the specially suited homoeopathic medicine can scarcely be prepared too small to effect perceptible amelioration in the disease for which it is appropriate (§§ 275-278), we should act injudiciously and hurtfully were we when no improvement, or some, though it be even slight, aggravation ensues, to repeat or even increase the dose of the same medicine, as is done in the old system, under the delusion that it was not efficacious on account of its small quantity (its too small dose). Every aggravation by the production of new symptoms – when nothing untoward has occurred in the mental or physical regimen – invariably proves unsuitableness on the part of the medicine formerly given in the case of disease before us, but never indicates that the dose has been too weak.

[152] The well informed and conscientiously careful physician will never be in a position to require an antidote in his practice if he will begin, as he should, to give the selected medicine in the smallest possible dose. Like minute doses of a better chosen remedy will re-establish order throughout.

[153] As I have more particularly described in the introduction to "Ignatia" (in the first volume of the Materia Medica Pura).

[154] The signs of improvement in the disposition and mind, however, may be expected only soon after the medicine has been taken when the dose has been sufficiently minute (i.e., as small as possible), an unnecessary large dose of even the most suitable homoeopathic medicine acts too violently, and at first produces too great and too lasting a disturbance of the mind and disposition to allow us soon to perceive the improvement in them. I must here observe that this so essential rule is chiefly transgressed by presumptuous tryos in homoeopathy, and by physicians who are converted to homoeopathy from the ranks of the old school. From old prejudices these persons abhor the smallest doses of the lowest dilutions of medicine in such cases, and hence they fail to experience the great advantages and blessings of that mode of proceeding which a thousandfold experience has shown to be the most salutary; they cannot effect all that homoeopathy is capable of doing, and hence they have no claim to be considered its adherents.

[155] The softest tones of a distant flute that in the still midnight hours would inspire a tender heart with exalted feelings and dissolve it in religious ecstasy, are inaudible and powerless amid discordant cries and the noise of day.

[156] *Coffee; fine Chinese and other herb teas; beer prepared with medicinal vegetable substances unsuitable for the patient's state; so-called fine liquors made with medicinal spices; all kinds of punch; spiced chocolate; odorous waters and perfumes of many kinds; strong-scented flowers in the apartment; tooth powders and essences and perfumed sachets compounded of drugs; highly spiced dishes and sauces; spiced cakes and ices; crude medicinal vegetables for soups; dishes of herbs, roots and stalks of plants possessing medicinal qualities; old cheese, and meats that are in a state of decomposition, or that passes medicinal properties (as the flesh and fat of pork, ducks and geese, or veal that is too young and sour viands), ought just as certainly to be kept from patients as they should avoid all excesses in food, and in the use of sugar and salt, as also spirituous drinks, heated rooms, woollen clothing next the skin, a sedentary life in close apartments, or the frequent indulgence in mere passive exercise (such as riding, driving or swinging), prolonged suckling, taking a long siesta in a recumbent posture in bed, sitting up long at night, uncleanliness, unnatural debauchery, enervation by reading obscene books, subjects of anger, grief or vexation, a passion for play, over-exertion of*

the mind or body, especially after meals, dwelling in marshy districts, damp rooms, penurious living, etc. All these things must be as far as possible avoided or removed, in order that the cure may not be obstructed or rendered impossible. Some of my disciples seem needlessly to increase the difficulties of the patient's dietary by forbidding the use of many more, tolerably indifferent things, which is not to be commended.

[157] Coffee; fine Chinese and other herb teas; beer prepared with medicinal vegetable substances unsuitable for the patient's state; so-called fine liquors made with medicinal spices; all kinds of punch; spiced chocolate; odorous waters and perfumes of many kinds; strong-scented flowers in the apartment; tooth powders and essences and perfumed sachets compounded of drugs; highly spiced dishes and sauces; spiced cakes and ices; crude medicinal vegetables for soups; dishes of herbs, roots and stalks of plants possessing medicinal qualities; asparagus with long green tips, hops, and all vegetables possessing medicinal properties, celery, onions; old cheese, and meats that are in a state of decomposition, or that passes medicinal properties (as the flesh and fat of pork, ducks and geese, or veal that is too young and sour viands), ought just as certainly to be kept from patients as they should avoid all excesses in food, and in the use of sugar and salt, as also spirituous drinks, undiluted with water, heated rooms, woollen clothing next the skin, a sedentary life in close apartments, or the frequent indulgence in mere passive exercise (such as riding, driving or swinging), prolonged suckling, taking a long siesta in a recumbent posture in bed, sitting up long at night, uncleanliness, unnatural debauchery, enervation by reading obscene books, reading while lying down, Onanism or imperfect or suppressed intercourse in order to prevent conception, subjects of anger, grief or vexation, a passion for play, over-exertion of the mind or body, especially after meals, dwelling in marshy districts, damp rooms, penurious living, etc. All these things must be as far as possible avoided or removed, in order that the cure may not be obstructed or rendered impossible. Some of my disciples seem needlessly to increase the difficulties of the patient's dietary by forbidding the use of many more, tolerably indifferent things, which is not to be commended.

[158] This is, however, rare. Thus, for instance, in pure inflammatory diseases, where aconite is so indispensable, whose action would be destroyed by partaking of vegetable acids, the desire of the patient is almost always for pure cold water only.

[159] All crude animal and vegetable substances have a greater or less amount of medicinal power, and are capable of altering man's health, each in its own peculiar way. Those plants and animals used by the most enlightened nations as food have this advantage over all others, that they contain a larger amount of nutritious constituents; and they differ from the others in this that their medicinal powers in their raw state are either not very great in themselves, or are diminished by the culinary processes they are subjected to in cooking for domestic use, by the expression of the pernicious juice (like the cassava root of South America), by fermentation (of the rye-flour in the dough for making bread, sour-crout prepared without vinegar and pickled gherkins), by smoking and by the action of heat (in boiling, stewing, toasting, roasting, baking), whereby the medicinal parts of many of these substances are in part destroyed and dissipated. By the addition of salt (pickling) and vinegar (sauces, salads) animal and vegetable substances certainly lose much of their injurious medicinal qualities, but other disadvantages result from these additions.

But even those plants that possess most medicinal power lose that in part or completely by such processes. By perfect desiccation all the roots of the various kinds of iris, of the horseradish, of the different species or arum and the peonies lose almost all their medicinal virtue. The juice of the most virulent plants often becomes inert, pitch-like mass, from the heat employed in preparing the ordinary extracts. By merely standing a long time, the expressed juice of the most deadly plants becomes quite powerless; even at moderate atmospheric temperature it rapidly takes on the vinous fermentation (and thereby loses much of its medicinal power), and immediately thereafter the acetous and putrid fermentation, whereby it is deprived of all peculiar medicinal properties; the fecula that is then deposited, if well washed, is quite innocuous, like ordinary starch. By the transudation that takes place when a number of green plants are laid one above the other, the greatest part of their medicinal properties is lost.

[160] Buchholz (Taschenb. f. Scheidek. u. Apoth. a. d. J., 1815, Weimar, Abth. I, vi) assures his readers (and his reviewer in the Leipziger Literaturzeitung, 1816, No. 82, does not contradict him) that for this excellent mode of operating medicines we have to thank the campaign in Russia, whence it was (in 1812) imported into Germany. According to the noble practice of many Germans to be unjust towards their own countrymen, he conceals the fact that this discovery and those directions, which he quotes in my very words from the first edition of the Organon of Rational Medicine, § 230 and note, proceed from me, and that I first published them to the world two years before the Russian campaign (the Organon appeared in 1810). Some folks would rather assign the origin of a discovery to the deserts of Asia than to a German to whom the honor belongs. O tempora! O mores!

Alcohol has certainly been sometimes before this used for mixing with vegetable juices, e.g., to preserve them some time before making extracts of them, but never with the view of administering them in this form.

[161] Although equal parts of alcohol and freshly expressed juice are usually the most suitable proportion for affecting the deposition of the fibrinous and albuminous matters, yet for plants that contain much thick mucus (e.g. Symphytum officinale, Viola tricolor, etc.), or an excess of albumen (e.g., Aethusa cynapium, Solanum nigrum, etc.), a double proportion of alcohol is generally required for this object. Plants that are very deficient in juice, as Oleander, Buxus, Taxus, Ledum, Sabina, etc., must first be pounded up alone into a moist, fine mass and the stirred up with a double quantity of alcohol, in order that the juice may combine with it, and being thus extracted by the alcohol, may be pressed out; these latter may also when dried be brought with milk-sugar to the millionfold trituration, and then be further diluted and potentized (v. § 271)

[162] In order to preserve them in the form of powder, a precaution is requisite that has hitherto been usually neglected by druggists, and hence powders, even of well-dried animal and vegetable substances could not be preserved uninjured even in well-corked bottles. The entire crude vegetable substances, though perfectly dry, yet contain, as an indispensable condition of the cohesion of their texture, a certain quantity of moisture, which dose not indeed prevent the unpulverized drug from remaining in as dry a state as is requisite to preserve it from corruption, but which is quite too much for the finely pulverized state. The animal or vegetable substance which in its entire state was perfectly dry, furnishes, therefore, when finely pulverized, a somewhat moist powder, which without rapidly becoming spoilt and mouldy, can yet not be preserved in corked bottles if not previously freed from this superfluous moisture. This is the best effected by spreading out the powder in a flat tin saucer with a raised edge, which floats in a vessel full of boiling water (i.e. a water-bath), and, by means of stirring it about, drying it to such a degree that all the small atoms of it (no longer stick together in lumps, but) like dry, fine sand, are easily separated from each other, and are readily converted into dust. In this dry state the fine powders may be kept forever uninjured in well-corked and sealed bottles, in all their original complete medicinal power, without ever being in-

jured by mites or mould; and they are best preserved when the bottles are kept protected from the daylight (in covered boxes, chests, cases). If not shut up in air-tight vessels, and not preserved from the access of the light of the sun and day, all animal and vegetable substances in time gradually lose their medicinal power more and more, even in the entire state, but still more in the form of powder.

[163] Long before this discovery of mine, experience had taught several changes which could be brought about in different natural substances by means of friction, for instance, warmth, heat, fire, development of odor in odorless bodies, magnetization of steel, and so forth. But all these properties produced by friction were related only to physical and inanimate things, whereas it is a law of nature according to which physiological and pathogenic changes take place in the body's condition by means of forces capable of changing the crude material of drugs, even in such as had never shown any medicinal properties. This is brought about by trituration and succussion, but under the condition of employing an indifferent vehicle in certain proportions. this wonderful physical and especially physiological and pathogenic law of nature had not been discovered before my time. No wonder then, that the present students of nature and physicians (so for unknowing) cannot have faith in the magical curative powers of the minute doses of medicines prepared according to homoeopathic rules (dynamized).

[164] The same thing is seen in a bar of iron and steel where a slumbering trace of latent magnetic force cannot but be recognized in their interior. Both, after their completion by means of the forge stand upright, repulse the north pole of a magnetic needle with the lower end and attract the south pole, while the upper end shows itself as the south pole of the magnetic needle. But this is only a latent force; not even the finest iron particles can be drawn magnetically or held on either end of such a bar.

Only after this bar of steel is dynamized, rubbing it with a dull file in one direction, will it become a true active powerful magnet, one able to attract iron and steel to itself and impart to another bar of steel by mere contact and even some distance away, magnetic power and this in a higher degree the more it has been rubbed. In the same way will triturating a medicinal substance and shaking of its solution (dynamization, potentation) develop the medicinal powers hidden within and manifest them more and more or if one may say so, spiritualizes the material substance itself.

[165] On this account it refers to the increase and stronger development of their power to cause changes in the health of animals and men if these natural substances in this improved state, are brought very near to the living sensitive fibre or come in contact with it (by means of intake or olfaction). Just as a magnetic bar especially if its magnetic force is increased (dynamized) can show magnetic power only in a needle of steel whose pole is near or touches it. The steel itself remains unchanged in the remaining chemical and physical properties and can bring about no changes in other metals (for instance, in brass), just as little as dynamized medicines can have any action upon lifeless things.

[166] We hear daily how homoeopathic medicinal potencies are called mere dilutions, when they are the very opposite, i.e., a true opening up of the natural substances bringing to light and revealing the hidden specific medicinal powers contained within and brought forth by rubbing and shaking. The aid of a chosen, unmedicinal medium of attenuation is but a secondary condition.

Simple dilution, for instance, the solution of a grain of salt will become water, the grain of salt will disappear in the dilution with much water and will never develop into medicinal salt which by means of our well prepared dynamization, is raised to most marvellous power.

[167] In order to maintain a fixed and measured standard for developing the power of liquid medicines, multiplied experience and careful observation have led me to adopt two succussions for each phial, in preference to the greater number formerly employed (by which the medicines were too highly potentized). There are, however, homoeopathists who carry about with them on their visits to patients homoeopathic medicines in the fluid state, and who yet assert that they do not become more highly potentized in the course of time, but they thereby show their want of ability to observe correctly. I discovered a grain of soda in half an once of water mixed with alcohol in a phial, which was thereby filled two-thirds full, and shook this solution continuously for half an hour, and this fluid was in potency and energy equal to the thirtieth development of power.

[168] One-third of one hundred grains sugar of milk is put in a glazed porcelain mortar, the bottom dulled previously by rubbing it with fine, moist sand. Upon this powder is put one grain of the powdered drug to be triturated (one drop of quicksilver, petroleum, etc.). The sugar of milk used for dynamization must be of that special pure quality that is crystallized on strings and comes to us in the shape of long bars. For a moment the medicines and powder are mixed with a porcelain spatula and triturated rather strongly, six to seven minutes, with the pestle rubbed dull, then the mass is scraped from the bottom of the mortar and from the pestle for three to four minutes, in order to make it homogeneous. This is followed by triturating it in the same way 6 – 7 minutes without adding anything more and again scraping 3 – 4 minutes from what adhered to the mortar and pestle. The second third of the sugar of milk is now added, mixed with the spatula and again triturated 6 – 7 minutes, followed by the scraping for 3 – 4 minutes and trituration without further addition for 6 – 7 minutes. The last third of sugar of milk is then added, mixed with the spatula and triturated as before 6 -7 minutes with most careful scraping together. The powder thus prepared is put in a vial, well corked, protected from direct sunlight to which the name of the substance and the designation of the first product marked /100 is given. In order to raise this product to /10000, one grain of the powdered /100 is mixed with the third part of 100 grains of powdered sugar of milk and then proceed as before, but every third must be carefully triturated twice thoroughly each time for 6 -7 minutes and scraped together 3 -4 minutes before the second and last third of sugar of milk is added. After each third, the same procedure is taken. When all is finished, the powder is put in a well corked vial and labelled /10000, i.e., (I), each grain containing 1/1,000,000 the original substance. Accordingly, such a trituration of the three degrees requires six times six to seven minutes for triturating and six times 3 -4 minutes for scraping, thus one hour for every degree. After one hour such trituration of the first degree, each grain will contain 1/000; of the second 1/10,000; and in the third 1/1,000,000 of the drug used.* Mortar and spatula must be cleaned well before they are used for another medicine. Washed first with warm water and dried, both mortar and pestle, as well as spatula are then put in a kettle of boiling water for half an hour. precaution might be used to such an extent as to put these utensils on a coal fire exposed to a glowing heat.

   * These are the three degrees of the dry powder trituration, which if carried out correctly, will effect a good beginning for the dynamization of the medicinal substance.

[169] The vial used for potentizing is filled two-thirds full.
[170] Perhaps on a leather bound book.
[171] They are prepared under supervision by the confectioner from starch and sugar and the small globules freed from fine dusty parts by passing them through a sieve. Then they are put through a strainer that will permit only 100 to pass through weighing one grain, the most serviceable size for the needs of a homoeopathic physician.

[172] A small cylindrical vessel shaped like a thimble, made of glass, porcelain or silver, with a small opening at the bottom in which the globules are put to be medicated. They are moistened with some of the dynamized medicinal alcohol, stirred and poured out on blotting paper, in order to dry them quickly.

[173] According to first directions, one drop of the liquid of a lower potency was to be taken to 100 drops of alcohol for higher potentiation. This proportion of the medicine of attenuation to the medicine that is to be dynamized (100:1) was found altogether too limited to develop thoroughly and to a high degree the power of the medicine by means of a number of such succussions without specially using great force of which wearisome experiments have convinced me.

But if only one such globule be taken, of which 100 weigh one grain, and dynamize it with 100 drops of alcohol, the proportion of 1 to 50,000 and even greater will be had, for 500 such globules can hardly absorb one drop, for their saturation. With this disproportionate higher ratio between medicine and diluting medium many successive strokes of the vial filled two-thirds with alcohol can produce a much greater development of power. But with so small a diluting medium as 100 to 1 of the medicine, if many succussions by means of a powerful machine are forced into it, medicines are then developed which, especially in the higher degrees of dynamization, act almost immediately, but with furious, even dangerous violence, especially in weakly patients, without having a lasting, mild reaction of the vital principle. But the method described by me, on the contrary, produces medicines of highest development of power and mildest action, which, however, if well chosen, touches all suffering parts curatively.* In acute fevers, the small doses of the lowest dynamization degrees of these thus perfected medicinal preparations, even of medicines of long continued action (for instance, belladonna) may be repeated in short intervals. In the treatment of chronic diseases, it is best to begin with the lowest degrees of dynamization and when necessary advance to higher, even more powerful but mildly acting degrees.

* In very rare cases, notwithstanding almost full recovery of health and with good vital strength, an old annoying local trouble continuing undisturbed it is wholly permitted and even indispensably necessary, to administer in increasing doses the homoeopathic remedy that has proved itself efficacious but potenized to a very high degree by means of many succussions by hand. Such a local disease will often then disappear in a wonderful way.

[174] This assertion will not appear improbable, if one considers that by means of this method of dynamization (the preparations thus produced, I have found after many laborious experiments and counter-experiments, to be the most powerful and at the same time mildest in action, i.e., as the most perfected) the material part of the medicine is lessened with each degree of dynamization 50,000 times yet incredibly increased in power, so that the further dynamization of 125 and 18 ciphers reaches only the third degree of dynamization. The thirtieth thus progressively prepared would give a fraction almost impossible to be expressed in numbers. It becomes uncommonly evident that the material part by means of such dynamization (development of its true, inner medicinal essence) will ultimately dissolve into its individual spirit-like, (conceptual) essence. In its crude state therefore, it may be considered to consist really only of this underdeveloped conceptual essence.

[175] As is still more circumstantially described in the prefaces to Arsenic and Pulsatilla in the Materia Medica Pura.

[176] Until the State, in the future, after having attained insight into the indispensability of perfectly prepared homoeopathic medicines, will have them manufactured by a

competent impartial person, in order to give them free of charge to homoeopathic physicians trained in homoeopathic hospitals, who have been examined theoretically and practically, and thus legally qualified. The physician may then become convinced of these divine tools for purposes of healing, but also to give them free of charge to his patients – rich and poor.

[177] Some homoeopathists have made the experiment, in cases where they deemed one remedy homoeopathically suitable for one portion of the symptoms of a case of disease, and a second for another portion, of administering both remedies at the same time; but I earnestly deprecate such a hazardous experiment, which can never be necessary, though it may sometimes seem to be of use.

[178] These globules (§ 270) retain their medicinal virtue for many years, if protected against sunlight and heat.

[179] Two substances, opposite to each other, united into neutral Natrum and middle salts by chemical affinity in unchangeable proportions, as well as sulphurated metals found in the earth and those produced by technical art in constant combining proportions of sulphur and alkaline salts and earths, for instance (natrum sulph. and calcarea sulph.) as well as those ethers produced by distillation of alcohol and acids may together with phosphorus be considered as simple medicinal substances by the homoeopathic physician and used for patients. On the other hand, those extracts obtained by means of acids of the so-called alkaloids of plants, are exposed to great variety in their preparation (for instance, chinin, strychnine, morphine), and can, therefore, not be accepted by the homoeopathic physician as simple medicines, always the same, especially as he possesses, in the plants themselves, in their natural state (Peruvian bark, nux vomica, opium) every quality necessary for healing. Moreover, the alkaloids are not the only constituents of the plants.

[180] When the rational physician has chosen the perfectly homoeopathic medicine for the well-considered case of disease and administered it internally, he will leave to irrational allopathic routine the practice of giving drinks or fomentations of different plants, of injecting medicated glysters and of rubbing in this or the other ointment.

[181] The praise bestowed of late years by some few homoeopathists on the larger doses is owing to this, either that they chose low dynamizations of the medicines to be administered, as I myself used to do twenty years ago, from not knowing any better, or that the medicines selected were not perfectly homoeopathic.

[182] See note to §246.

[183] Let them learn from the mathematicians how true it is that a substance divided into ever so many parts must still contain in its smallest conceivable parts always some of this substance, and that the smallest conceivable part does not cease to be some of this substance and cannot possibly become nothing; – let them, if they are capable of being taught, hear from natural philosophers that there are enormously, powerful things (forces) which are perfectly destitute of weight, as, for example, caloric, light, etc., consequently infinitely lighter than the medicine contained in the smallest doses used in homoeopathy; – let them, if they can, weigh the irritating words that bring on a bilious fever, or the mournful intelligence respecting her only son that kills the mother; let them touch, for a quarter of an hour, a magnet capable of lifting a hundred pounds weight, and learn from the pain it excites that even imponderable agencies can produce the most violent medicinal effects upon man; – and let the weak ones among them allow the pit of the stomach to be slightly touched by the thumb's point of a strong-willed mesmeriser for a few minutes, and the disagreeable sensations they then suffer will

make them repent of attempting to set limits to the boundless activity of nature; the weak-minded creatures!

If the allopathist who is trying the homoeopathic system imagine he cannot bring himself to give such small and profoundly attenuated doses, let him only ask himself what risk he runs by so doing? If the scepticism which holds what is ponderable only to be real, and all that is imponderable to be nothing, be right, nothing worse could result from a dose that appears to him to be nothing, than that no effect would ensue – and consequently this would be always much more innocuous than what must result from his too large doses of allopathic medicine. Why will he consider his inexperience, coupled with prejudice, more reliable than an experience of many years corroboration by facts? And, moreover, the homoeopathic medicine becomes potentized at every division and diminution by trituration or succussion! – a development of the inherent powers of medicinal substances which was never dreamed of before my time, and which is of so powerful a character that of late I have been compelled by convincing experience to reduce the ten succussions formerly directed to be given after each attenuation, to two.

[184] The rule to commence the homoeopathic treatment if chronic diseases with the smallest possible doses and only gradually to augment them is subject to a notable exception in the treatment of the three great miasms while they still effloresce on the skin, i.e., recently erupted itch, the untouched chancre (on the sexual organs, labia, mouth or lips, and so forth), and the figwarts. These not only tolerate, but indeed require, from the very beginning large doses of their specific remedies of ever higher and higher degrees of dynamization daily (possibly also several times daily). If this course be pursued, there is no danger to be feared as is the case in the treatment of diseases hidden within, that the excessive dose while it extinguishes the disease, initiates and by continued usage possible produces a chronic medicinal disease. During external manifestations of these three miasms this is not the case; for from the daily progress of their treatment it can be observed and judged to what degree the large dose withdraws the sensation of the disease from the vital principle day by day; for none of these three can be cured without giving the physician the conviction through their disappearance that there is no longer any further need of these medicines.

Since diseases in general are but dynamic attacks upon the life principle and nothing material – no materia peccans – as their basis (as the old school in its delusion has fabulated for a thousand years and treated the sick accordingly to their ruin) there is also in these cases nothing material to take away, nothing to smear away, to burn or tie or cut away, without making the patient endlessly sicker and more incurable (Chron. Dis. Part 1), than he was before local treatment of these three miasms was instituted. The dynamic, inimical principle exerting its influence upon the vital energy is the essence of these external signs of the inner malignant miasms that can be extinguished solely by the action of a homoeopathic medicine upon the vital principle which affects it in a similar but stronger manner and thus extracts the sensation of internal and external spirit-like (conceptual) disease enemy in such a way that it no longer exists for the life principle (for the organism) and thus releases the patient of his illness and he is cured.

Experience, however, teaches that the itch, plus its external manifestations, as well as the chancre, together with the inner venereal miasm, can and must be cured only by means of specific medicines taken internally. But the figwarts, if they have existed for some time without treatment, have need for their perfect cure, the external application of their specific medicines as well as their internal use at the same time.

[185] Supposing one drop of a mixture that contains 1/10 of a grain of medicine produces an effect = a; one drop of a more diluted mixture containing 1/100th of a grain of the medicine will only produce an effect = a/2; if it contain 1/10000th of a grain of medicine, about = a/4; if it contain 1/100000000th of a grain of medicine it will produce and effect = a/8; and thus it goes on, the volume of the doses being equal, with every (perhaps more than) quadratic diminution of the quantity of medicine, the action on the human body will be diminished each time to only about one-half. I have very often seen a drop of the decillion-fold dilution of tincture of nux vomica produce pretty nearly just half as much effect as a drop of the quintillion-fold dilution, under the same circumstances and in the same individual.

[186] The power of medicines acting upon the infant through the milk of the mother or wet nurse is wonderfully helpful. Every disease in a child yields to the rightly chosen homoeopathic medicines given in moderate doses to the nursing mother and so administered, is more easily and certainly utilized by these new world-citizens than is possible in later years. Since most infants usually have imparted to them psora through the milk of the nurse, if they do not already possess it through heredity from the mother, they may be at the same time protected antipsorically by means of the milk of the nurse rendered medicinally in this manner. But the case of mothers in their (first) pregnancy by means of a mild antipsoric treatment, especially with sulphur dynamizations prepared according to the directions in this edition (§ 270), is indispensable in order to destroy the psora – that producer of most chronic diseases – which is given them hereditarily; destroy it both within themselves and in the foetus, thereby protecting posterity in advance. This is true of pregnant women thus treated; they have given birth to children usually more healthy and stronger, to the astonishment of everybody. A new confirmation of the great truth of the psora theory discovered by me.

[187] For this purpose it is most convenient to employ fine sugar globules of the size of poppy seeds, one of which imbibed with the medicine and put into the dispensing vehicle constitutes a medicinal dose, which contains about the three hundredth part of a drop, for three hundred such small globules will be adequately moistened by one drop of alcohol. The dose is vastly diminished by laying one such globule alone upon the tongue and giving nothing to drink. If it be necessary, in the case of a very sensitive patient, to employ the smallest possible dose and to bring about the most rapid result, one single olfaction merely will suffice (see note to §288).

[188] From this fact may be explained those marvellous cures, however infrequent, where chronic deformed patients, whose skin nevertheless was sound and clean, were cured quickly and permanently after a few baths whose medicinal constituents (by, chance) were homoeopathically related. On the other hand, the mineral baths very often brought on increased injury with patients, whose eruptions on the skin were suppressed. After a brief period of well-being, the life principle allowed the inner, uncured malady to appear elsewhere, more important for life and health.

At times, instead, the ocular nerve would become paralyzed and produce amaurosis, sometimes the crystalline lens would become clouded, hearing lost, mania or suffocating asthma would follow or an apoplexy would end the sufferings of the deluded patient.

A fundamental principle of the homoeopathic physician (which distinguishes him from every physician of all older schools) is this, that he never employs for any patient a medicine, whose effects on the healthy human has not previously been carefully proven and thus made known to him (§§ 20,21). To prescribe for the sick on mere conjecture of some possible usefulness for some similar disease or from hearsay "that a remedy has helped in such and such a disease" – such conscienceless venture the philanthropic homoeopathist will leave to the allopath. A genuine physician and practitioner or our art will therefore never send the sick to any of the numerous mineral baths, because almost all are unknown so far as their accurate, positive effects on the healthy human organism is concerned, and when misused, must be counted among the most violent and dangerous drugs. In this way, out of a thousand sent to the most celebrated of these baths by ignorant physicians allopathically uncured and blindly sent there perhaps one or two are cured by chance more often return only apparently cured and the miracle is proclaimed aloud. Hundreds, meanwhile sneak quietly away, more or less worse and the rest remain to prepare themselves for their eternal resting place, a fact that is verified by the presence of numerous well-filled graveyards surrounding the most celebrated of these spas.*

* A true homoeopathic physician, one who never acts without correct fundamental principles, never gambles with the life of the sick entrusted to him as in a lottery where the winner is in the ratio of 1 to 500 or 1000 (blanks here consisting of aggravation or death), will never expose any one of his patients to such danger and send him for good luck to a mineral bath, as is done so frequently by allopaths in order to get rid of the sick in an acceptable manner spoiled by him or others.

[189] It is only the most simple of stimulants, wine and alcohol, that have their heating and intoxicating action diminished by dilution with much water.

[190] By the word intimately I mean this: that when, for instance, the drop of a medicinal fluid has been shaken up once with one hundred drops of spirits of wine; that is to say, the phial containing both, held in the hand, has been rapidly moved from above downwards with a single smart jerk of the arm, there certainly ensues a thorough mixture of the whole, but with two, three, ten and more such strokes, this mixture becomes much more intimate; that is to say, the medicinal power becomes much more potentized, and the spirit of this medicine, so to speak, becomes much more unfolded, developed and rendered much more penetrating in its action on the nerves. If, then, the required object we wish to attain with the low dilutions be the diminution of the doses for the purpose of moderating their powers upon the organism, we would do well to give no more than two such succussion-jerks to each of the twenty, thirty, etc., dilution phials, and thus to develop the medicinal power only moderately. It is also advisable, in attenuating the medicine in the state of dry powder by trituration in a porcelain mortar, to keep within certain limits, and, for example, to triturate strongly, for one hour only, one grain of the crude entire medical substance, mixed with the first hundred grains of milk-sugar (to the 1/10000th attenuation) likewise only for one hour, and to make the third attenuation (to 1/1000000) also by one hour of strong trituration of one grain of the previous mixture with one hundred grains of milk-sugar, in order to bring the medicine to such an attenuation that its development of power shall remain moderate. A more exact description of this process will be found in the prefaces to Arsenic and Pulsatilla in the Materia Medica Pura.

[191] The higher we carry the attenuation accompanied by dynamization (by two succussion strokes), with so much the more rapid and penetrating action does the preparation seem to affect the vital force and to alter the health, with but slight diminution of strength even when this operation is carried very far, – in place, as is usual (and generally sufficient) to X when it is carried up to XX, L, C, and higher; only that then the action always appears to last a shorter time.

[192] It is especially in the form of vapour, by olfaction and inhalation of the medicinal aura that is always emanating from a globule impregnated with a medicinal fluid in a high development of power, and placed, dry, in a small phial, that the homoeopathic remedies act most surely and most powerfully. The homoeopathic physician allows the

patient to hold the open mouth of the phial first in one nostril, and in the act of inspiration draw the air out of it into himself and then if he wished to give a stronger dose, smell in the same manner with the other nostril, more or less strongly, according to the strength it is intended the dose should be, he then corks up the phial and replaces it in his pocket case to prevent any misuse of it, and unless he wishes it he has no occasion for an apothecary's assistance in his practice. A globule of which ten, twenty or one hundred weigh one grain, impregnated with the thirtieth potentized dilution, and then dried, retains for this purpose all its power undiminished for at least eighteen or twenty years (my experience extends this length of time), even though the phial be opened a thousand times during that period, if it be but protected from heat and the sun's light. Should both nostrils be stopped up by coryza or polypus, the patient should inhale by the mouth, holding the orifice of the phial betwixt his lips. In little children it may be applied close to their nostrils whilst they are asleep with the certainty of producing an effect. The medicinal aura thus inhaled comes in contact with the nerves in the walls of the spacious cavities it traverses without obstruction, and thus produces a salutary influence on the vital force, in the mildest yet most powerful manner, and this is much preferable to every other mode of administering the medicament in substance by the mouth. All that homoeopathy is capable of curing (and what can it not cure beyond the domain of mere manual surgery affections?) among the most severe chronic diseases that have not been quite ruined by allopathy, as also among acute disease, will be most safely and certainly cured by this olfaction. I can scarcely name one in a hundred out of the many patients that have sought the advice of myself and my assistant during the past year, whose chronic or acute disease we have not treated with the most happy results, solely by means of this olfaction; during the latter half of this year, moreover, I have become convinced (of what I never could previously have believed) that by this olfaction the power of the medicines is exercised upon the patient in, at least, the same degree of strength, and that more quietly and yet just as long as when the dose of medicine is taken by the mouth, and that, consequently, the intervals at which the olfaction should be repeated should not be shorter than in the ingestion of the material dose by the mouth.

[193] Especially of one of such persons, of whom there are not many, who, along with great kindness of disposition and perfect bodily powers, possesses but a very moderate desire for sexual intercourse, which it would give him very little trouble wholly to suppress, in whom, consequently, all the fine vital spirits that would otherwise be employed in the production of the semen, are ready to be communicated to others, by touching them and powerfully exerting the will. Some powerful mesmerisers, with whom I have become aquatinted, had all this peculiar character.

[194] A patient even destitute of the sense of smell may expect an equally perfect action and cure from the medicine by olfaction.

[195] When I here speak of the decided and certain curative power of positive mesmerism, I most assuredly do not mean that abuse of it, where, by repeated passes of this kind, continued for half an hour or a whole hour at a time, and, even day after day, performed on weak, nervous patients, that monstrous revolution of the whole human system is effected which is termed somnambulism, wherein the human being is ravished from the world of sense and seems to belong more to the world of spirits – a highly unnatural and dangerous state, by means of which it has not infrequently been attempted to cure chronic diseases.

[196] It is a well known rule that a person who is either to be positively or negatively mesmerised, should not wear silk on any part of the body.

[197] Hence a negative pass, especially if it be very rapid, is extremely injurious to a delicate person affected with a chronic ailment and deficient in vital force.

[198] A strong country lad, ten years of age, received in the morning, on account of slight indisposition, from a professed female mesmeriser, several very powerful passes with the points of both thumbs, from the pit of the stomach along the lower edge of the ribs, and he instantly grew deathly pale, and fell into such a state of unconsciousness and immobility that no effort could arouse him, and he was almost given up for dead. I made his eldest brother give him a very rapid negative pass from the crown of the head over the body to the feet, and in one instance he recovered his consciousness and became lively and well.

[199] Rubbing-in appears to favour the action of the medicines only in this way, that the friction makes the skin more sensitive, and the living fibres thereby more capable of feeling, as it were, the medicinal power and of communicating to the whole organism this health-affecting sensation. The previous employment of friction to the inside of the thigh makes the mere laying on the mercurial ointment afterwards quite as powerfully medicinal as if the ointment itself had been rubbed upon that part, a process which is termed rubbing-in, but it is very doubtful whether the mental itself can penetrate in substance into the interior of the body, or be taken up by the absorbent vessels by means of this so-called rubbing-in. Homoeopathy, however, hardly ever requires for its cures the rubbing-in of any medication, nor does it need any mercurial ointment.

[200] The smallest homoeopathic dose, which however, often effects wonders when used on proper occasions. Imperfect homoeopathists, who think themselves monstrously clever, not infrequently deluge their patients in difficult diseases with doses of different medicines, given rapidly one after the other, which, although they may have been homoeopathically selected and given in highly potentized attenuation, bring the patients into such an over-excited state that life and death are struggling for the mastery, and the least additional quantity of medicine would infallibly kill them. In such cases a mere gentle mesmeric pass and the frequent application, for a short time of the hand of a well-intentioned person to the part that is particularly affected, produce the harmonious uniform distribution of the vital force throughout the organism, and therewith rest, sleep and recovery.

[201] Although by this restoration of the vital force, which ought to be repeated from time to time, no permanent cure can be effected in cases where, as has been taught above, a general internal dyscrasia lies at the root of the old local affection, as it always does, yet this positive strengthening and immediate saturation with the vital force (which no more belongs to the category of palliatives than does eating and drinking when hunger and thirst are present) is no mean auxiliary to the actual treatment of the whole disease by homoeopathic medicines.

[202] Especially of one of those persons, of whom there are not many who, along with great kindness of disposition and perfect bodily powers, possesses but a very moderate desire for sexual intercourse, which it would give him very little trouble to suppress, in whom, consequently, all the fine vital spirits that would otherwise be employed in the preparation of the semen, are ready to be communicated to others, by touching them and powerfully exerting the will. Some powerful mesmerisers, with whom I have become acquainted, has all this peculiar character.

[203] When I here speak of the decided and certain curative power of positive mesmerism, I most assuredly do not mean the abuse of it, where, by repeated passes of this kind, continued for half an hour or a whole hour at a time, and, even day after day, performed on weak, nervous patients, that monstrous revolution of the whole human sys-

tem is effected which is termed somnambulism, wherein the human being is ravished from the world of sense and seems to belong more to the world of spirits – a highly unnatural and dangerous state, by means of which it has not infrequently been attempted to cure chronic diseases.

[204] It is a well known rule that a person who is either to be positively or negatively mesmerised, should not wear silk on any part of the body.

[205] Hence a negative pass, especially if it be very rapid, is extremely injurious to a delicate person affected with a chronic ailment and deficient in vital force.

[206] A strong country lad, ten years of age, received in the morning, on account of slight indisposition, from a professed female mesmeriser, several very powerful passes with the points of both thumbs, from the pit of the stomach along the lower edge of the ribs, and he instantly grew pale, and fell into such a state of unconsciousness and immobility that no effort could arouse him, and he was almost given up for dead. I made his eldest brother give him a very rapid negative pass from the crown of the head over the body to the feet, and in one instant he recovered his consciousness and became lively and well.

Made in the USA
Lexington, KY
09 September 2019